"George Roth is a talented and intuitive hands-on clinician. Much of clinical practi[illegible] do it because it works. Roth goes beyond that. He devours information like a spider eating its prey, organizes it, and then spins it out in a complex web that enmeshes theory and practice in a highly developed system. The Matrix concept builds on the structural concept of biotensegrity, in which the bony skeleton is enmeshed in a highly structured soft tissue matrix, and integrates it with proven therapeutic musculoskeletal medical techniques drawn from his clinical armamentarium. He has been able to simplify the system so that it is easily explainable, readily teachable, and now, with this book, widely available. Here is a simple mechanical method for diagnosing and safely treating a variety of musculoskeletal malfunctions that will be useful for clinicians and also as a self-help book for those dealing with persistent structural impairments. This is not a cure-all for everything that ails you but a specific treatment method for specific problems. It tells you how to find them and how to treat them. Try it."

—Stephen Levin, MD
Orthopedic surgeon, former associate clinical professor at Michigan State University in East Lansing, MI, and former assistant clinical professor of orthopedic surgery at Howard University in Washington, DC

"My practice is based on seeing patients who have not achieved success with traditional treatment. They often come to see me as a last resort. I have been using Matrix Repatterning for four years on a variety of diagnoses, from sports injuries to painful joints to chronic pain. I have been very excited about the results, seeing significant functional improvement and pain reduction in just a few visits. I encourage my colleagues and the public to look into this breakthrough program."

—Debora Hickman, MS, PT Physical therapist and doctoral candidate of physical therapy at Loma Linda University in Loma Linda, CA

"I am a strong advocate of Matrix Repatterning, and I whole-heartedly endorse it for everybody. It makes a lot of sense once it is understood. I know that every training room and major pro team will be using Matrix Repatterning in the future because it works better than anything out there, and as athletes, we are results driven. Matrix Repatterning delivers!"

—Mark Cunningham
Athlete and personal coach

"I am the mother of four very active children. They have constant bumps and falls (skating, bicycling, and so forth). Matrix Repatterning has allowed us to overcome many of these injuries with the tools we have learned. I can hardly imagine how our family ever managed without it. Thank you so much for this amazing program."

—B.L.
Mother of four and Matrix Repatterning Program adherent

The Matrix Repatterning Program *for* Pain Relief

SELF-TREATMENT FOR MUSCULOSKELETAL PAIN

GEORGE ROTH, DC, ND

New Harbinger Publications, Inc.

Publisher's Note

This publication is designed to provide accurate and authoritative information in regard to the subject matter covered. It is sold with the understanding that the publisher is not engaged in rendering psychological, financial, legal, or other professional services. If expert assistance or counseling is needed, the services of a competent professional should be sought.

Distributed in Canada by Raincoast Books

New Harbinger Publications
5674 Shattuck Avenue
Oakland, CA 94609

Photographs by Matthew Wiley
Illustrations by Jeanne Robertson
Cover design by Amy Shoup
Acquired by Melissa Kirk
Text design by Tracy Marie Carlson

ISBN 1-57224-391-0 Paperback

Printed in the United States of America

New Harbinger Publications' Web site address: www.newharbinger.com

07 06 05

10 9 8 7 6 5 4 3 2 1

First printing

This book is dedicated to the thousands of patients I have had the privilege of treating over the course my 26 years in practice to date. They have been my supreme motivation to achieve excellence. Many have become friends and all have taught me the value of pursuing the truth at the heart of the human condition. I honor them for their courage to explore this new field of medicine with me, and for providing me with so many insights, on a daily basis, which inspire my work.

When one tugs at a single thing in Nature, he finds it hitched to the rest of the Universe.

—John Muir

The patterns within us,
Charged with life.
Universal—infinitesimal,
From protons to planets.
All of Nature—one fabric,
bound together.

—George B. Roth

Contents

Foreword

Dr. George Roth is an internationally known practitioner and teacher who has dedicated himself to gathering new insights into the healing process. His clients come from around the globe, seeking help for conditions that have stumped the best of therapists. Over the years, Dr. Roth and his students have perfected a systematic approach to painful conditions that can be used by anyone. In his seminars, he has demonstrated to many people that they can resolve many of their aches and pains and even treat themselves.

Nearly all therapeutic traditions recognize that the human body, and not the doctor, is responsible for the healing process. Within limits, our bodies have all of the powers needed to resolve our bumps and bruises, aches and pains. All a therapist can do is give the system a helpful push to start the healing process when it has stalled for whatever reason.

We still have doctors because we have somehow lost touch with our built-in healing mechanisms. Sooner or later, though, someone was going to do what Dr. Roth has now done: discover and reveal basic techniques of self-treatment all of us can use. Fortunately George writes with a clear and engaging style that enables us to quickly grasp and practice the ideas he and his colleagues have spent years developing.

In this book, Dr. Roth treats us to a vision of the human body as a highly efficient and successful system with enormous powers of self-regulation. The key to his therapeutic success is a recognition that the body is made of a continuously interconnected matrix that obeys certain simple rules. To know and use these rules is to be delivered from both pain and the fear that often comes with it.

Matrix Repatterning is vital for the athlete or performer, as well as the average person, striving for new levels of accomplishment and well-being, while reducing chances of reinjury. But it also has a message our whole culture urgently needs. The ways we have been taught to react to pain are a disaster. We have been repeatedly told that pain and other symptoms are enemies—messengers that are to be killed before giving us any news of what is taking place within us. We do not have time for pain, and are bombarded daily with new ways of chasing it away, usually without addressing the cause. In this manner we thwart the wisdom of our bodies, harm ourselves even more, and postpone the healing process.

Matrix Repatterning is a far more mature approach to pain and symptoms in general. It is an approach that honors the biological processes our bodies use to get our attention. For those suffering from acute or chronic pain, such as from fibromyalgia or repetitive motion disorders, the book is worth reading just for the demystification it brings to a profoundly important part of our biology. Demystification is vital, for pain and misplaced fear of what it signifies can drastically inhibit the healing process.

Of key importance is the rule that the place that hurts is often not the real source of the problem. So Dr. Roth provides us with simple and effective methods for learning the truth of the messages coming from our bodies. And then he reveals gentle ways of allowing tissues to remember their normal structure and function. The methods employ our own energy, a profound built-in healing force that we have been discouraged from thinking about, let alone utilizing on our own. The work of repatterning can be done while we go about our daily activities, and can "turn the clock back" by resolving layer after layer of old trauma. Many people are going to feel a lot more comfortable and happy in their bodies as a result of the methods described here.

This is a book that many of us have been waiting for. There are lots of important writings on therapeutic technique, but few if any that show the average person how to heal themselves. Thank you, George, for your dedication to humanity and your passionate generosity of spirit that shine from every page of this book.

—James L. Oschman, Ph.D.
Dover, New Hampshire
October 2004

Acknowledgments

There are so many who have influenced and inspired me to write this book and to develop this method. The following deserve special recognition.

It has been said that we all stand on the shoulders of those who have come before us. Dr. Stephen Levin, orthopedic surgeon and pioneer of the tensegrity structural concept, has been a friend and mentor for many years. His landmark discoveries and insights have opened a vast new horizon of possibility for me as a clinician. His energy and enthusiasm are an inspiration to everyone interested in the pursuit of truth. I value his wisdom and look forward to our continuing association as teachers and researchers in this exciting field.

Dr. Donald Ingber, a noted cell biologist at Harvard Medical School, has verified for the world the foundational concepts of tensegrity at the cellular level. His work has served to open new vistas into the realm of medicine in general and the structural concepts that I continue to explore.

There have been many inspiring and enlightening influences from the field of health care: Dr. John Upledger, Dr. Harold Schwartz, Dr. Lawrence Jones, Dr. Paul Chauffour, Dr. Jean-Pierre Barral, Dr. Edgar Houle, Dr. Herbert Lee, to name a few. Dr. James Oschman, the author of *Energy Medicine: The Scientific Basis*, has provided us with many amazing insights into the scientific foundation of manual therapy and the healing process. He has also been invaluable with his help in editing the final manuscript.

There are also numerous students and colleagues who continue to provide valuable insights and inspiration: Kim Clarke, R.N., R.M.T., Dr. Barbara Brown, Evelyn Barton, P.T. and Debbie Hickman, P.T., to name a few. Many of them have struggled with me through the numerous evolutionary changes in the development of these concepts and their clinical application. Thanks to Dr. Scott Kircher for his wonderful analogy of the plastic water bottle to demonstrate the effect of treatment.

I wish to thank my agent Arnold Gosewich for taking a chance on me, and for his calm professionalism. The staff at New Harbinger, including Melissa Kirk, Carole Honeychurch, and Heather Mitchener, have kept me on track and provided useful assistance in the editing and organization of this work. I want to thank Matthew Wiley, friend and gifted photographer, and Jeanne Robertson, an equally gifted illustrator, both of whom had worked on my previous book, *Positional Release Therapy*. They have shown the utmost patience in the sometimes difficult task of developing the visual material for this book. Special thanks to my dear niece Jana Shapero, for being the model for the self-treatment section. Thanks to Kim and her delightful children Matthew and Emily for their support and being models for the Treating Children section. I also wish to thank my dedicated staff, Edna McNair and Penny Foster, for their continuing support, and keeping me honest over the years.

I especially want to thank my family, including my sons Joshua and Noah, for the joy and richness they add to my life.

Introduction

We human beings are indeed marvels. Our bodies are beautifully designed to express well-being and the fullness of life. Unfortunately, when you are in pain, the idea of enjoying the fullness of life may seem out of reach. Often, what you may read about the subject of pain or have been told by health practitioners only adds to your confusion and distress. The aim of this book is to provide you with a sound basis of fact and a clearer understanding of health based on how the body is actually put together. Knowledge is power, and understanding how the body works and the amazing degree to which it is a self-regulating and self-healing mechanism can serve to allay much of the fear associated with health conditions as they arise.

Even though this book's title mentions pain relief, it will become clear as you read on why pain itself is never the real issue. Pain is merely an uncomfortable message the body provides when it's in distress. It is not appropriate to kill the messenger. The message is that something is out of balance. The key is to find out where it's coming from and what is wrong.

Matrix Repatterning could be the key to discovering what is wrong and where it is in the body. It addresses imbalances within the structure of the body at the molecular level—imbalances that often go undetected by traditional methods. It has been found that the body thrives when the molecular structure, forming the cells of every part of the body, is in balance (Ingber 1998). Organ function, breathing,

Limiting beliefs are based on fear. Pain is amplified by the fear of the unknown. I believe that when we understand the nature of how we are made and how we can easily overcome many of the structural imbalances affecting our health, we will be able to rise above our limitations and achieve a new level of awareness and well-being.

digestion, muscle tone, sleep patterns, and even one's state of mind—all of these seem to benefit when the layers of tension are released gently and effectively through the methods described in this book.

THE SEARCH FOR ANSWERS

I have been engaged in the study of health and disease for over twenty-five years. In the course of my training, I had been taught there was a connection between the structure of the body and its function. I believed that the way we were put together had a purpose, and that in order for everything to work properly, the structure of the body needed to be in balance.

I studied various methods of treatment supposedly designed to restore balance to the body and soon discovered that the theories being taught didn't always deliver their promised results. My impression was that most methods were ultimately ineffective in creating any significant changes. I knew I had to keep searching. In the words of the illustrious physicist, Dr. Richard P. Feynman: "If the theory does not fit the facts, then the theory must be wrong" (Feynman 1974).

Finally, I found a few basic principles that seemed promising. Some of these came from the fields of chiropractic and osteopathy. These are forms of manipulation of the body developed in the late nineteenth century. I was especially influenced by certain practitioners and teachers who were cutting-edge, out-of-the-box thinkers. Despite the fact that I was achieving an increasing level of success, I still could not explain the successes or the failures. There were as many theories as there were techniques, and none of them could adequately explain how they were affecting the body.

THE LIGHTS GET TURNED ON: THE TENSEGRITY MATRIX REVEALED

Gradually, the direct application of these structural theories began to emerge. My clinical experiences became more focused, and I was gradually able to translate these into a coherent and consistent assessment and treatment process. What finally evolved was the overall approach described in this book.

In 1993, I met Dr. Stephen Levin, an orthopedic surgeon and founder of the Potomac Back Center in Vienna, Virginia. We were both teaching at a physical medicine conference at York University in Toronto. In 1977 Dr. Levin had come up with a radical theory that the body was actually composed of microscopic, molecular subunits forming a continuous geodesic framework. He used the term *tensegrity*, a word coined by Buckminster Fuller, the famous engineer and architect. Fuller had theorized back in the 1940s that this structure, made from a continuous network of tension and compression elements, was the most efficient way to make buildings and, indeed, was likely the way most structures in nature were constructed. Fuller became famous for building large geodesic buildings based on these concepts.

When I first met Levin, the basic research to establish tensegrity as the basis of organic life had not yet been published. But as soon as I heard him speak, I knew this was it! Here, finally, was a theory that seemed to fit the facts. Dr. Levin had not developed a clinical method for applying these principles, but I instinctively knew that tensegrity could potentially be my own missing link, a foundation for understanding some of my own observations and clinical experience.

Dr. Levin and I began discussing the implications of tensegrity in the field of physical medicine. He was able to clarify how the tensegrity molecular framework could easily account for the responses in the assessment and treatment procedures I had been developing. All of the confusing, conflicting concepts I had struggled with were suddenly beginning to align within the framework of this one, powerful unifying theory. It was as if the pieces in a huge, complex jigsaw puzzle were beginning to fall into place of their own accord.

Before being exposed to the concept of tensegrity, I felt as if I had been walking down a dark tunnel, taking one cautious step forward at a time, feeling for the solid ground beneath my feet. Now, it was as if the entire tunnel were lit up with brilliant light. I could see for miles ahead. Instead of my tenuous progress, I was suddenly able to sprint forward at top speed. Having a solid concept of how things were actually put together allowed me to extrapolate my clinical experience to every possible level within the body with greater confidence.

In recent years, research by scientists such as Donald E. Ingber, M.D., Ph.D., a Harvard-based cell biologist, has proven the existence of this molecular framework inside each cell, right down to the level of the DNA (genetic material inside each cell). I refer to this structure as the *tensegrity matrix* or simply the *matrix*. These discoveries have helped to explain many of the mechanical properties displayed by the body and have expanded our understanding of how the mechanics of the cell are related to health and disease.

Gradually, the direct application of these structural theories began to emerge. My clinical experiences became more focused, and I was gradually able to translate these into a coherent and consistent assessment and treatment process. What finally evolved was the overall approach described in this book. The goal of Matrix Repatterning is to restore or repattern the natural state of balance at the molecular/cellular level, the matrix. Matrix Repatterning is a comprehensive system based on sound scientific principles that can help alleviate many painful conditions and health problems associated with structural imbalance. The treatment normalizes the structural effects of physical injury and allows the body to be restored to its normal, balanced pattern and optimum function.

MEETING THE CHALLENGE

I had been teaching small groups of practitioners (chiropractors, physical therapists, sports medicine specialists, massage therapists, and even some veterinarians), but I eventually realized that I needed to do more. I had to get the message out to regular folks, real people in real pain. I knew if I could somehow communicate some of these basic truths, it might help to dispel a lot of the fear and discouragement associated with back pain and other physical conditions. I felt strongly that it could help them regain a sense of their own power in the face of their pain and alleviate many of the other problems caused by structural imbalance, problems that limited their ability to experience the fullness of life.

Over the years since I first began to develop some these concepts and techniques, my colleagues and I have seen results that have amazed us. I am continually awed by the power of the universal principles unerringly expressed in the human form. The tensegrity matrix *is* the structural basis of all life on the planet. Noted scientists have now proven this fact (Duncan 1995; Heidemann 1993; Ingber 1998; Wang, Butler, and Ingber 1993). I had uncovered truths that I and my colleagues and students have been able to consistently reproduce. We were able to demonstrate the primary sources of tension—the source of structural imbalance leading to pain—that other trained practitioners could confirm consistently.

Many of my previous belief systems were being challenged and exposed by the truth of the principles I was discovering. I could no longer believe that bone is rigid, that hardened (fibrotic) muscle requires endless deep-tissue massage, that spinal curvatures are cast in stone, or that any part of the body is separate from any other part. All of these beliefs were being shattered and so was my limited understanding of what could be treated and restored to its original state of balance and optimal function.

The challenge, of course, has been to make these principles accessible to everyone. Combined with an understanding of how the tensegrity matrix governs our structure and function, I wanted to find a way to provide the average person in pain with simple tools to alleviate some of the effects of injury at the deep, cellular/molecular level. The program described in this book is my attempt to achieve this goal. But healing is an art, and it is not reasonable to expect that these techniques can replace the need for professional attention in all cases. However, the program presented in this book can provide you with the tools you need to overcome many day-to-day injuries and strains. It may also provide you with relief from some chronic pain issues. It can also give you hope—the hope that these concepts can offer a solution to help you return to the joyful, pain-free life you intend to live.

AN INVITATION

I invite you to join the many people around the world who have experienced the benefits of Matrix Repatterning in this liberating journey of self-discovery.

You can become an active participant in your own health care through the self-help program provided in this book and through choosing health-care practitioners, when needed, to help you easily and gently overcome more challenging conditions. The purpose of Matrix Repatterning is to normalize and support the capacity of every part of the body to function at its optimal level. It is my experience that when the body tissues are restored to their ideal level of tone and balance, they are able to withstand tremendous forces and resist the tendency to become seriously injured in the first place.

This book will provide you with practical tools to help restore your body to an optimal level of function and relieve many painful musculoskeletal conditions. The Matrix Repatterning Program will provide you with a simple and effective method to assess and treat your own body, along with guidelines to help you determine if your situation requires the intervention of a health-care professional. In addition to these techniques, you will learn a simple exercise program to help you stay in balance and therefore reduce your tendency to become injured in the first place.

My hope is that the Matrix Repatterning Program will alleviate much unnecessary suffering. Once we become aware of the potential of our bodies to heal easily and quickly and how Matrix Repatterning can restore balance to the molecular structure, it will be easier for us to relax and allow health and well-being to become our expectation. Cells are the basis of every tissue in the body, and since cells are being normalized through this process, every part of the body can benefit. This may be why such an apparently wide range of conditions appears to respond to this approach.

The body has a tremendous capacity to heal itself. When the cells of the body have access to their full potential, they are capable of resisting many illnesses and recovering from illness once it develops. We are not passive receptacles of disease. We do have the ability to rally significant resources to help us live long, healthy, and productive lives. Matrix Repatterning and the self-treatment methods described in this book can be an important ally in restoring our capacity for self-healing and the maintenance of optimal health.

CHAPTER 1

Breakthrough

It was during one of our sessions, after we had released one of her more stubborn problems, that she grabbed my hand. Heather looked up at me and announced in a deliberate tone, quavering with intensity: "You have to teach this. To everyone!"

Heather's Story: A New Lease on Life

Heather arrived at my office, a look of disdain on her face. She didn't seem to notice the homey touches: the plants, the fireplace, much less the pleasant sunny summer day outside. She was on a mission. She was here to see yet another practitioner who would undoubtedly fail her. Heather had been in constant pain for twenty-eight of her thirty-four years. At six years of age she had fallen twenty feet out of a ski lift. Typical of this feisty lady, she had landed on her feet. Unfortunately, her little body could not support the force of her landing. Her legs and pelvis were smashed and she began a new life, one that would see her endure numerous surgeries and hospitalizations, not to mention constant, agonizing pain.

Heather suffered from pain in her head, neck, shoulders, upper back, lower back, hips, and legs. She had limited movement in her hips and legs and experienced dizziness, digestive problems, and reproductive disorders, including a lack of sensation in her pelvis. She had sought help for many years from physical therapists, chiropractors, bodyworkers, acupuncturists, and psychologists, all to no avail.

Despite all of this, she had pursued a challenging career as a biologist, one that would see her engage in daunting wilderness treks and primitive camping expeditions. She continued to ski and even worked as a white-water rafting outfitter. She sustained numerous subsequent injuries from these exploits, which of course aggravated her condition. Heather had made the decision to tackle life for all it was worth. She dared life to try and deny her the experiences she felt were her right. She was a fighter. And yet, she carried her pain with her wherever she went. It tempered her confidence and limited her more adventurous pursuits and her joy.

She had read about my work and had decided to give me a try. But after all the treatment options she had tried unsuccessfully, she couldn't help being skeptical. She was angry—angry at the world and at the many practitioners who had claimed they could provide help but had consistently disappointed her. One tiny part of her still wanted to believe there was something out there that could help, but the fear of more disappointment held that slender hope in check.

I explained the basis of Matrix Repatterning and the scientific evidence for the structural theory behind it. Her background in biology gave me the opportunity to wax eloquent on the elegant theories behind the approach I had developed.

Following our first session, she mentioned that her pelvis felt more free and perhaps less painful. I reminded her that she still had a long way to go and that her long history of fairly serious injuries would be revealed in layers. However, despite all my caveats, I felt fairly confident that we would succeed where others had failed.

Well, as you might have guessed, "Pride goeth before a fall." When she came into the consultation room on her next visit a week later, Heather looked like she had her own personal rain cloud following her around. I had explained, during our first session, that a brief aggravation of symptoms, lasting one to three days, was not unusual. This represented a reawakening of the pain pathways that the brain had adapted to over time. Well, she had indeed experienced an aggravation, and it hadn't gone away in a few days as promised. She was in a lot of pain in several new areas, and her pelvis felt worse than ever! My bubble burst, and I acknowledged that I needed to dig deeper to uncover more of her underlying problems.

To make a long story short, Heather, like many of my most difficult cases, provided a tremendous learning opportunity. On the basis of what I discovered in her case, I was subsequently able to help many other people with serious injuries due to falls. Eventually, after a series of sessions and a lot of effort on both our parts, Heather began to turn the corner. She noticed her hips were able to move more normally, and she could turn her head without agony. Her digestive system began to function normally. She expressed to me that she felt more in her body.

It was during one of our sessions, after we had released one of her more stubborn problems, that Heather grabbed my hand. She looked up at me and announced in a deliberate tone, quavering with intensity: "You have to teach this. To everyone!"

I was humbled by the power of Heather's declaration. In that moment, I became fully aware of all of the pain she had resolutely endured for so many years. And I knew then the extent of the gift that Matrix Repatterning represented. I had known that this process was able to create real changes in people's bodies, but suddenly I was struck by the difference it could make in people's lives.

WHAT IS THE MATRIX?

When you studied science at school, you may have been taught that the cell is a bag of fluid with stuff floating around inside. However, in the mid 1970s it was discovered that each cell contained a molecular framework, referred to as the *cytoskeleton.* This is a sort of molecular scaffold composed of microscopic protein filaments. The cytoskeleton determines the shape and mechanical properties of the cell. If the cell is mechanically compressed or stretched, the shape of the cytoskeleton will be altered, and the effects of these changes will be transmitted throughout the cell immediately. It has been demonstrated that changes in tension and shape of the cytoskeleton have a significant effect on how the cell functions (Ingber 1998; Hatfaludy, Hannsky, and Vandenburgh 1989; Ko, Arora, and McCulloch 2001).

In addition to this, binding proteins on the cell membrane connect each cell to every other cell, forming a continuous fabric throughout the body ("the hip bone's connected . . ."). This interconnected framework within each cell and between cells is what I have termed the tensegrity matrix or simply the matrix. The matrix is now the established basis for the molecular structure of the entire body and for all life on the planet. It explains how cells and the whole body move, respond to mechanical forces, and utilize nutrients and energy. The matrix has been shown to have very specific mechanical and electronic properties that have a significant influence on health and disease. Leading researchers are beginning to recognize its implications in everything from heart disease to cancer (Ingber 1998, 2002; Ko, Arora, and McCulloch 2001; Masi and Walsh 2003).

The matrix is amazingly resilient and allows us to perform all kinds of activities, from housework to walking to competing in the Olympics. It is even capable of bouncing back into shape when significant forces are applied to it. The flexible matrix allows us to withstand a significant amount of force without any ill effects. But there is a limit. Sometimes there are forces that are just too much for our structure to absorb.

When we experience a significant strain or fall or get into a fender bender (or worse), the molecules that make up the matrix may become locked into a rigid pattern (see figure 1-1 below).

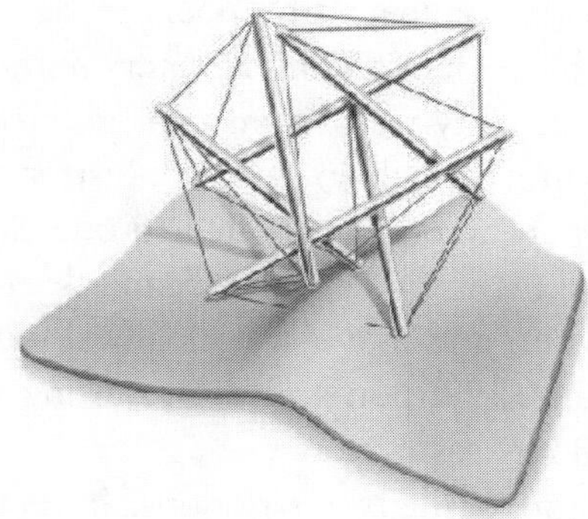

Neutral, relaxed
molecular state

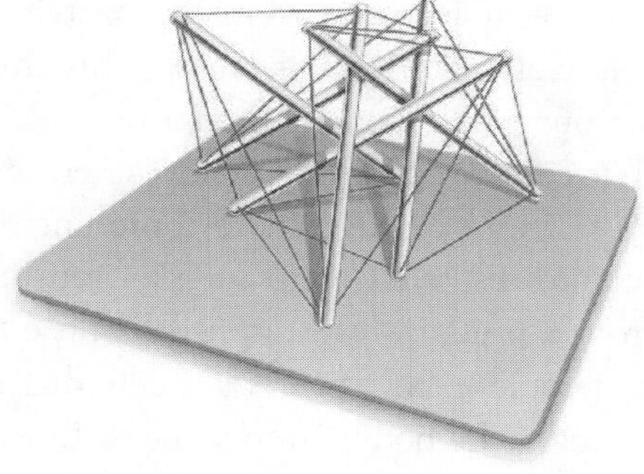

Strained, rigid
molecular state

Figure 1-1: Normal and strained tensegrity structure
Based on "The Architecture of Life" *Scientific American,* Jan. 1998.

SCIENCE CONFIRMS THE TENSEGRITY MATRIX

Inside every cell of the body there are a series of thousands of tiny cables and struts made of protein (actin and myosin). Together, these protein strands form a framework providing the cell with certain properties such as strength and flexibility. Donald Ingber and many other have provided the hard scientific proof of the existence of this structure. A very useful resource is the book by Dr. James Oschman, *Energy Medicine: The Scientific Basis* (2000). His book details the properties of the body, including the tensegrity matrix, and how these relate to health and the healing process.

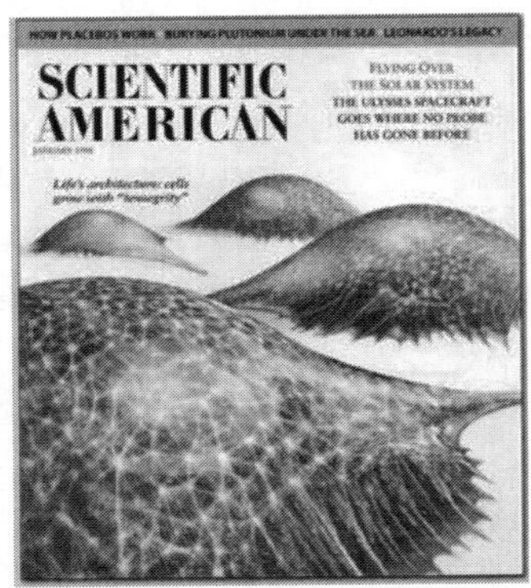

Figure 1-2:
"The Architecture of Life"
Reprinted with permission.

The principles of tensegrity apply at essentially every detectable size scale in the human body. . . . Thus, from the molecules to the bones and muscles and tendons of the human body, tensegrity is clearly nature's preferred building system. Only tensegrity, for example, can explain how every time that you move your arm, your skin stretches, your extracellular matrix extends, your cells distort, and the interconnected molecules that form the internal framework of the cell feel the pull—all without any breakage or discontinuity.

—Donald E. Ingber, M.D., Ph.D.,*
"The Architecture of Life"

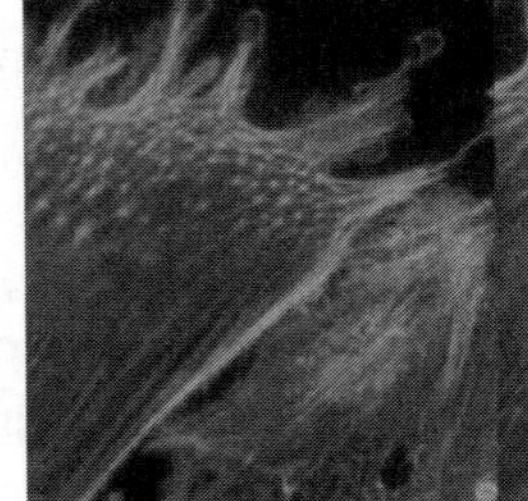

Figure 1-3: Cytoskeleton showing tensegrity structure
Sui Huang, M.D., Ph.D. and Don Ingber, M.D., Ph.D.

HOW WE GET OUT OF BALANCE: THE PRIMARY RESTRICTION

The matrix is generally very flexible and incredibly strong. When significant force is applied to it by injuries such as severe strain or impact, it can absorb some of this force or energy. This in turn alters the arrangement of molecules within the protein fibers. When this happens, the fibers in the area of injury become relatively rigid (Ingber 1998). This creates what we have identified as a *primary restriction.*

Since our whole body is interconnected, one or more primary restrictions can produce a pattern of tension that can extend throughout the entire body (see figure 1-4 below). In this illustration, the model is wearing a stretchy body suit to represent the matrix. When a corner is pulled to one side, the whole fabric becomes distorted, with lines of tension radiating from the pulled area. Similarly, the pattern of tension from a primary restriction will cause the body to strain and move abnormally. Much of the pain that many people experience is actually due to this transmitted tension and the resulting strain created in other parts of the body, often some distance from the primary restriction.

With subsequent injuries and the development of more primary restrictions, layer upon layer of tension is added and the matrix becomes more and more restricted. In addition, an area that already contains a primary restriction is less flexible than normal tissue. Therefore, subsequent injuries will tend to be absorbed by this area to a greater degree and create a larger area of restriction. As the matrix goes further out of balance, there is an increasing likelihood of strain and pain from seemingly minor injuries.

* Dr. Ingber does not formally endorse the Matrix Patterning approach.

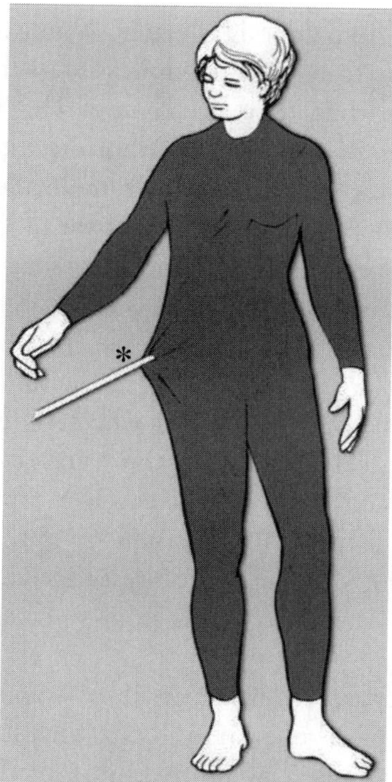

Figure 1-4: Strain patterns from one primary restriction*

* Reprinted from *Positional Release Therapy* 1997, with permission from Elsevier.

FACTORS AFFECTING THE MATRIX

The human frame is unique in the animal world, primarily due to our upright, standing posture. We have also introduced an array of technological innovations that tend to put us in harm's way: the automobile, high-speed and contact sports, and heavy equipment in industrial settings, to name a few. We are prone to certain illnesses due to lifestyle choices such as poor diet and sedentary activities. Exposure to chemical toxins and various forms of radiation may impact on the cells of our body as well. Surgical scarring and even the dentist's drill—as we will discover below—may also result in primary restrictions. In addition, the demands and stresses of daily life in this highly technological era can have a negative influence on our overall level of health.

Mechanical Factors

The matrix is capable of withstanding tremendous forces and loads due its inherent strength and resilience. However, forces beyond a certain threshold may be absorbed by the proteins forming the cellular scaffold.

There are two major forms of physical injury: strain and impact. Contact sports and injuries such as falls and car accidents are the most common sources of impact injury. Based on the laws of physics, the more dense the substance, the more mechanical energy it will absorb from an impact. This is because the molecules in a dense structure are closer together, which causes the force of the impact to be easily transferred from molecule to molecule. A less dense material will not transfer as much energy, instead dissipating most of the force of impact. For example, when you bang your knuckles on a table, you hear the distinctive sound vibrating back to your ear. This is because the molecules in the table are close together, which gives it its hardness. The energy of your knock is immediately transmitted from molecule to molecule and converted to sound energy that you can hear. Doing the same on a pillow, with its relatively less dense structure, will result in very little if any sound being created. This is also why protective equipment such as a helmet has a soft inner layer of foam—so that the force of impact will be dissipated before it reaches the wearer's head.

All living things on the planet—from viruses to vertebrates, plants to people—have been found to have the same basic structure. This is composed of an incredibly strong and flexible molecular network called the tensegrity matrix. It makes possible such seemingly impossible feats as the mobility of a giraffe's neck, the soaring flight of an eagle, and the contortions of an acrobat.

You may be surprised to learn that the most dense substance in the human body is water. Water is, in fact, one of the densest substances on earth. It is sometimes referred to as a noncompressible substance, meaning that its molecules cannot be pushed any closer together than they already are. This is why when you drop a balloon filled with water, it will explode. The energy of the impact is transferred to the water molecules inside the balloon, which convert it to movement. Since the water molecules cannot move closer together or inward, they move in the only way possible for them to go—outward.

The human body is 70 percent water. Much of this is in the blood vessels and in other spaces between cells where it can easily move around without any hindrance. However, there are certain areas where water is contained and cannot easily disperse. The large, fluid-filled organs like the heart, liver, spleen, and kidneys are similar in some ways to a water balloon. They are recognized by medicine as being extremely vulnerable to impact injury. You may have heard of people in car accidents who suffered a ruptured spleen. This is not necessarily due to a direct injury to the spleen, but simply the transfer of the force of the impact to the dense internal organs. If the force is sufficient, it will cause a rapid outward movement of the water molecules inside the organ. This sudden internal expansion leads to a direct transfer of the force of injury to the organ itself, as well as other surrounding structures. In severe cases, the organ may literally explode, leading to serious complications and even death from so-called internal injuries.

Another often-overlooked area of impact injury involves another very dense substance—bone. Structural changes in bone have often been associated with the process of degeneration due to arthritis. However, our own clinical research suggests that these changes may be caused by injury, and that the degenerative processes are actually initiated by these changes in the shape of the bone.

Strain is an overstretching of tissues and may involve muscles, ligaments, or joints. The body has a significant amount of elasticity and a built-in tolerance to strain. It is only when the force is severe or if the part that is strained has lost some of its elastic properties that the force of the strain is absorbed into the tissues, creating a permanent change in the molecular structure.

Scar tissue is produced by the body to replace damaged cells and tissues. It is usually composed of dense bundles of cells surrounded by relatively inelastic fibers. It may be produced by disease processes such as inflammation, from severe injury causing tissue damage, or from surgery. By definition, scar tissue is less elastic than normal tissue and therefore usually results in the formation of a primary restriction.

Electromagnetic Factors

The matrix, like all molecular structures, has specific structural and electrical properties. Figure 1-1 illustrates the two states in which the molecules making up the matrix can exist. The normal, relaxed state and the strained, rigid state have different arrangements of the protein filaments and the molecules within them. As a result, they may have slightly different electrical fields. Another way of stating this is that each molecular state has a different frequency, much like the different frequencies on a radio tuner. Albert Szent-Gyorgyi, the Nobel laureate for his discovery of vitamin C, is cited for his remarkable work showing how the body's proteins actually act as semiconductors, storing electrical charge and allowing electrical current to be conducted throughout the body (Szent-Gyorgyi 1977). This feature of the matrix is one of the concepts we use in the Matrix Repatterning assessment process, which will be discussed in chapter 4.

The properties of the matrix imply that its structure and its electrical state are interconnected. The normal flexible state appears to produce one electrical field or frequency, while the strained, rigid state appears to produce another frequency. As a result, the matrix may be affected by external sources of electromagnetic radiation.

Several studies (Liburdy et al. 1993; Burr 1972) have demonstrated a potential link between exposure to electrical fields and the development of disease. Matrix Repatterning practitioners have found that chronic exposure to strong artificial or *geopathic* (generated from within the earth) sources of electromagnetic radiation may have deleterious effects on the structural characteristics of the matrix and on general health. Identifying these sources of electrical influence is an important facet of determining the cause of certain disease processes. Potential sources of disturbing electromagnetic fields include transmission towers and transformers, household appliances, industrial equipment, and personal electronic equipment. Due to the conductive properties of metals, certain personal articles such as underwire bras and metal wristwatch bands may also interfere with the electrical balance of the body. Methods for assessing and addressing some of these influences are discussed in appendix 2.

Chemical Factors

The human body is 70 percent water by volume and water is critical to every physiological process both inside and outside the cell. Recently, water has been determined to exist in a specifically structured state within all life forms (Pollack 2001). Perhaps not surprisingly, this structure is in the form of a tensegrity matrix. Therefore the matrix is surrounded by water molecules within each cell. This combined form is the basis of the structural and functional integrity of the body.

We live in a world of chemicals. The food we eat, the air we breath, the dissolved elements in the water we drink continually bathe our cells, inside and out, with a host of nutrients, minerals, toxins, and pollutants. It is the job of various organs and systems to process, utilize, or dispose of these chemicals in the quest to maintain health and balance within the body. Various factors determine the efficiency of these systems and their capacity to cope with the multitude of chemical compounds to which they are exposed. Incomplete processing or inefficient waste disposal may result in the accumulation of toxic waste materials in the tissues of the body. The overexposure to toxic chemicals, heavy metals, or drug compounds may also lead to a toxic overload of the body. Many of these materials become lodged within the tissue fluids (as well as the molecules of the matrix) that bathe and surround the structural framework of the body.

A complex chemical interaction between these compounds and the fluids surrounding the matrix can lead to changes in viscosity (flexibility) of the extracellular and intracellular fluids and therefore the mechanical properties of the cellular matrix itself. An accumulation of these chemicals may affect the matrix, leading to a greater tendency to absorb the force of an injury or altering the body's ability to respond to corrective measures.

Thought and Emotion

As previously mentioned, the matrix has electronic and structural properties. Our thoughts and feelings generate electrical (as well as chemical) messages, which are, in turn, transmitted throughout the matrix. This is why stressful thoughts may lead to increased muscle tension and pain, while meditation and other forms of mental relaxation are helpful in relieving many physical conditions.

THE SOLUTION

Matrix Repatterning is a process of assessing and treating the structure of the body based on the underlying properties of the tensegrity matrix. It utilizes the unique mechanical and electrical properties of the matrix to gently restore balanced tone to the molecular structure.

Current research points to a strong connection between the structural and mechanical integrity of the body and its ability to function at an optimal level (Ingber 2003; Ko, Arora, and McCulloch 2001). The concept of the tensegrity matrix has been verified by a significant amount of scientific study (Wang, Butler, and Ingber 1993; Ingber 1998). It is the way the body is constructed, right down to the level of the cell and everything in between. It may be the basis of how the body responds to various influences, including injury, and therefore it may determine how the body responds—or does not respond—to various therapies.

The area of the primary restriction is often painless soon after the original injury (see chapter 3), while the parts of the body attempting to compensate for the primary problem may become strained and painful. Many therapies directed to the site of pain are therefore relatively ineffective in correcting the underlying problem. This is why so many painful conditions seem to reoccur or are simply resistant to these therapies.

As outlined above, injury—strain or impact—appears to have very specific mechanical and electronic effects on the molecular/cellular structure of the body. Any therapy, in order to be truly effective, may need to address this aspect of the response to injury. Therefore, the benefit of any form of treatment is likely due to its influence on the matrix. In general, forceful techniques tend to be less effective in creating change, since the very nature of the matrix is that it tends to resist forceful deformation. This may be due to the powerful electronic forces controlling its shape. In his research, Oschman has found that the most effective therapies are the ones that are the least forceful (2000).

Many forms of hands-on therapy may influence the matrix, depending on where the treatment is applied. This may be due to the normalizing electrical field in the therapist's hands. Therapies like massage, myofascial therapy, Rolfing, chiropractic, osteopathy, and similar approaches may owe at least part of their benefits to this factor. This may also explain the positive benefits of treatments in which direct touch is not employed. Therapeutic touch and similar "energy" techniques employ the use of off-the-body placement of the hands. It may be the normal electrical field in the hand that influences a shift toward normal in the injured area. Trigger-point therapy and acupuncture employ the use of direct stimulation of irritable focal points on the body. These may have the effect of causing a discharge of the stored electrical charge within the tissues, thus allowing a return to the neutral, relaxed state of the molecular structure. Positional Release Therapy also uses tender points on the surface of the body to guide the positioning of the body to release the stored tension in the primary restriction (D'Ambrogio and Roth 1997). Certain forms of exercise like yoga, tai chi, Feldenkrais, and the Alexander technique may work by placing the body in specific positions that allow for a release of the local area of tension in the area of primary involvement.

Matrix Repatterning views the body as an interconnected whole. The concept of the tensegrity matrix may explain how any one part of the body can affect any other part. The entire body is therefore assessed for possible primary restrictions. The location of symptoms is largely ignored, because it is understood that the key to restoring normal function depends on correcting the primary restrictions. Therefore, all of the information needed to restore the structure of the body to its ideal state of balance appears to be recorded within the body itself. The method for locating primary restrictions (Matrix Repatterning Self-Assessment) is described in chapter 4. You may discover that symptoms of low-back pain may even originate from a tooth, while the tension resulting in headaches may be coming from a restriction in one of the bones in the lower leg. As far-fetched as this sounds, these are surprisingly common findings. Gentle treatment at the source of the problem will then allow the body to balance itself and get back to doing what it does so well—thrive and express well-being.

The discovery of the tensegrity matrix has opened up a whole new way of understanding how the body is put together and how it may respond to injuries. Since cellular structure and function appear to depend on the mechanics of the matrix, these discoveries also provide us with new insights into the way the body expresses health and disease. When we truly understand how the body works, much of the fear and anxiety over painful physical conditions can be overcome. The discovery of the tensegrity matrix highlights the inherent resilience and stability of our structure and its apparent ability to be easily restored to its original balanced and functional condition.

The goal of Matrix Repatterning is to find and correct primary restrictions and ultimately to restore balance to the body. Although pain relief is not the purpose of this technique, it is usually achieved rather quickly and efficiently due to the reduction of strain and the restoration of normal tone to the tissues of the body. Matrix Repatterning provides us with a gentle and effective tool to restore the structural integrity of the body at the molecular level. It represents a radical departure from many of the limited and limiting beliefs that have pervaded the field of physical medicine. There is a new awareness that life exists and expresses itself in an integrated manner, a direct reflection of the underlying stuff of the universe from which we are all created and the indwelling intelligence that animates all that is. The principles and properties of the tensegrity matrix may explain how we respond to our environment, gravity, injuries, and the very processes governing health and disease.

Practitioners using Matrix Repatterning have found that many previously difficult cases, including most musculoskeletal conditions such as headache, back pain, neck pain, shoulder pain, hip pain, knee pain, carpal tunnel, frozen shoulder, and scoliosis, as well as certain types of digestive problems, heart conditions, reproductive disorders, and many other health concerns have responded favorably to this form of therapy. In most cases, the treatment period is brief, and the treatments themselves are painless. Many elite athletes have discovered that Matrix Repatterning is helping them recover from injuries that would have been considered career-ending by most other health professionals. Thoroughbred racehorses are also getting a new lease on life and performing beyond previous expectations thanks to the application of these principles in their therapy. Most people find it difficult to believe that treatments this gentle can have such profound effects on the body. Matrix repatterning is a concept that demystifies our experience of pain. This demystification itself can be a huge factor in healing by taking away fear, which can actually inhibit the healing process. And now you, too, can have the tools to help yourself. The Matrix Self-Treatment Program and the Matrix Exercise Program will provide you with practical and effective ways of dealing with many painful and limiting conditions, as well as promoting optimal health.

STRUCTURAL IMBALANCE: KEY POINTS

- The tensegrity matrix is the scientifically proven structure of all life on the planet. According to this new concept, the entire body (bones, muscles, organs, everything) is one continuous piece of fabric.
- The matrix provides stability and flexibility and absorbs energy from injuries and other sources.
- A significant force (strain or impact) may cause the molecules within the matrix to change to a rigid state and form a primary source of restriction.
- Dense structures such as internal organs (full of dense water) and bones absorb most of the energy in impact injuries and often become primary sources of restriction.
- Joints, muscles, and ligaments are designed to give way when strained but may form primary restrictions when overstretched. Scar tissue may also be a source of restriction.
- Strain patterns from the primary restrictions may cause many other parts of the body to move and function abnormally, resulting in pain and other health problems.
- Various influences (physical, electrical, chemical, and emotional) may influence the matrix, making it more susceptible to injury and more resistant to correction.

CHAPTER 2

What Is Matrix Repatterning?

Sarah was a thirty-two-year-old housewife who had been suffering from low back pain for over a year. After inviting her into my consultation room I asked about her history. She told me she had been very active in sports, including volleyball and figure skating, in her teenage years, and had sustained the usual falls and strains associated with her active lifestyle. She had two young children, one of whom had been born two years before by Cesarean section. She had been experiencing low back pain "for years" on and off, but the year before she had fallen on the steps from her back porch, landing on her rear end. Since then, the pain had not subsided, despite numerous physical therapy and chiropractic treatments.

Matrix Repatterning is a gentle and effective tool to restore the structural integrity of the body at the molecular level. It represents a radical departure from many of the limited and limiting beliefs that have pervaded the field of physical medicine. There is a new awareness that life exists and expresses itself in an integrated manner, a direct reflection of the underlying stuff of the universe from which we are all created and the indwelling intelligence that animates all that is. The principles and properties of the tensegrity matrix determine how we respond to our environment, gravity, injuries, and the very processes governing health and disease.

APPRECIATING PAIN

I began by telling her I was not concerned with getting rid of her pain. I waited the usual couple of beats for the shock of this statement to register.

I stated that I was solely interested in improving the function of her body. I told her that pain was the least reliable way to determine where her problem was coming from or what was needed to correct her body's structural balance. Simply getting rid of pain was not necessarily in her best interest.

"In fact," I said, "pain could save your life!" I went on to say that pain tells you that something, somewhere is wrong. It can warn you that moving a certain way or exerting yourself beyond a certain limit could threaten the integrity of the body tissues—joints, ligaments, muscles, or even a vital structure like an organ, a nerve, or the spinal cord itself. Damage to one of these structures could permanently impair your ability to feed yourself, escape a dangerous situation, or even to reproduce. Nature has designed this important feedback system to protect the species from extinction.

What pain does not tell you, however, is *where* the source of the problem is or even what is wrong. I stated that anyone can get rid of pain. If you want to get rid of a headache, for example, simply hit yourself on the toe with a hammer! It's so easy to fool the brain, where symptoms such as pain are generated.

CLOSE ENCOUNTER OF THE MATRIX REPATTERNING KIND

"Sit up straight, please," I suggested. I pushed down on her right shoulder. There was very little movement. Then I placed my other hand lightly over her lower ribs on the left. I pushed on her shoulder again, and this time it moved downward with ease. She looked at me, and I could see the typical expression: mouth and eyes wide open. She had just had her first encounter of the Matrix Repatterning kind!

"What was that?" she exclaimed.

I went on to explain the new theories about the tensegrity matrix and how this model explains many of the structural and electrical properties of the body, which science simply had no way of accounting for previously. I explained that Matrix Repatterning is based on a newly confirmed model for how the body is put together. "Researchers have discovered that within each cell there is a molecular scaffold made of proteins. We also know that the matrix of the body connects every part of the body to every other part, like a continuous sheet of fabric.

"The tensegrity matrix is a framework with very specific mechanical properties that seem to be the key to understanding what happens when we get injured. When we get injured, it is the fibers in the matrix that absorb the force of the strain. When that happens, the molecules inside the cells in that area change from a flexible state to one that is rigid. This creates something we call a primary restriction. Think of the primary restriction as a source of tension that is constantly putting all of the fibers of your body into a state of tension." I took hold of one corner of my sweater and pulled it to one side. "This area of restriction pulls on the rest of the body," I said, pointing to the strain lines in the fabric of the sweater leading to my opposite shoulder and neck. "Because of this source of tension, my neck and shoulder would tend to move abnormally and become strained." She nodded in understanding. "Now, if I could locate and release the primary restriction," I said pointing to the part of the sweater I was pulling, "and release it," I let go of the sweater, allowing the fabric to be restored to its more balanced shape, "it would reduce the strain on these other areas." That seemed to make sense to her.

I then showed Sarah a wood and elastic model representing the basic structure of the tensegrity matrix. I demonstrated the inherent flexibility of the three-dimensional structure by pushing and pulling at it from various angles (figure 2-1 below).

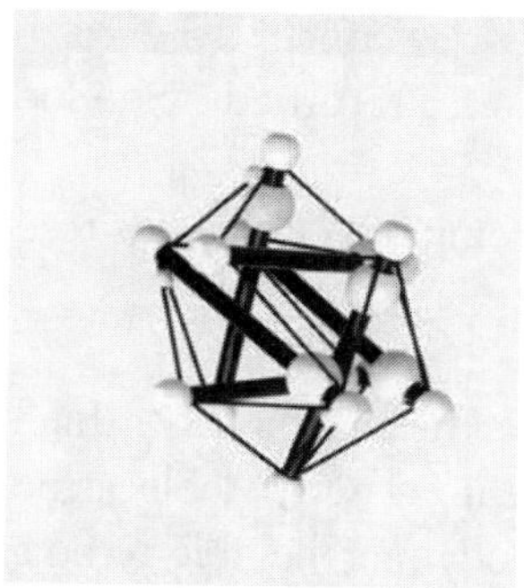

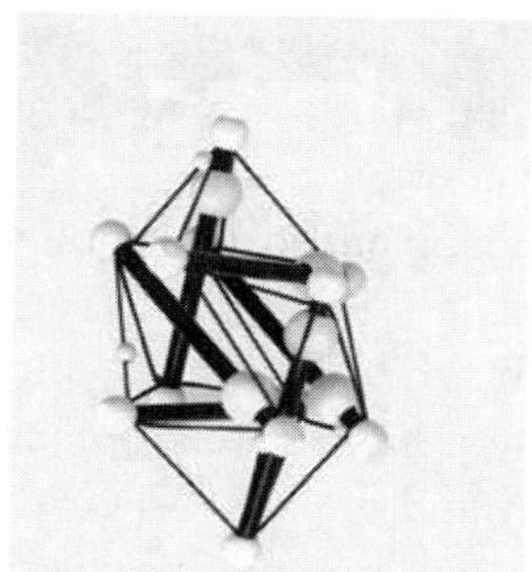

Figure 2-1: Neutral and strained tensegrity model

"This is the normal, relaxed state of the matrix that forms the molecular structure inside each cell of your body," I said holding the model in front of me without applying any strain to it, but gently pushing it from different directions to demonstrate its flexibility. "But if there is a significant strain or impact, as in a fall, this structure will absorb the force of the injury like this." I pulled the model from two ends so that it extended outward and became noticeably rigid. "This is called the strained state of the tensegrity matrix. The energy of the injury is absorbed by the molecule, which causes the whole structure to shift to a more rigid form. And this is where it gets stuck. It cannot get back to the normal state on its own."

SING THE BODY ELECTRONIC

"What happened when you put your hand on my lower ribs?"

"Well," I answered, "when the molecules shift, they seem to have a different arrangement of atoms and therefore they appear to produce a different electrical field or *electronic signature*, which, simply put, means that the molecules have changed to a new frequency."

"Oh, you mean like on my radio?"

"Yes, very much the same." I continued. "The strained, rigid molecules appear to be transmitting a frequency that's different from the surrounding normal, flexible ones. We know that when two different electrical fields are brought close together, they tend to influence each other. That's the same thing that happens when you bring two tuning forks close to each other. If one is vibrating, it will set another one with the same frequency potential into a synchronous vibration. Similarly, when I place my hand over an area of abnormal electronic pattern, the normal electrical field in my hand seems to influence the electrical field of the injured area toward a more normal frequency. Since the electrical field and the structure of the molecules are interrelated, the rigid molecules in the area seems to relax a bit as they return to a more normal shape. Since all the molecules in the body—bones, muscles, organs, and every cell—are interconnected like a continuous sheet of fabric, when the molecules in the primary area of injury relax as I place my hand over them, the whole body relaxes a little."

"And that's why my shoulder relaxed when you put your hand over my lower ribs. Your hand caused the injury—the restriction—in my ribs to become more normal. Is that it?"

"That's exactly it," I answered, amazed how well she grasped these new concepts.

"But then when you took your hand away, the tension in my shoulder returned." She looked at me in a rather perplexed way.

"Yes, the relaxing effect of placing my hand over the area is only temporary. It seems to take a little more energy to fully correct the pattern of tension."

"But why can't the body just heal itself?" she asked.

"It took quite a bit of force to cause the injury in the first place. The matrix has a high degree of tolerance to strain and impact. When there is a shift, it appears to create a new, stable arrangement of the molecules that will stay that way without some outside help. The body may be able to adapt to these abnormal patterns, up to a point. We can compensate for them because most of our structure is still relatively normal. With time and an accumulation of injuries however, our structure can go seriously out of balance," I pointed out.

LOOKING DEEPER FOR THE SOURCE

"In your case," I continued, "the bones and joints in your pelvis and your right kidney are the main sources of tension, or the primary restrictions, causing the rest of your body to be out of balance."

She looked puzzled. "Kidney? Why would my kidney be a problem? My doctor never told me I had a problem there."

"I don't mean that you have kidney disease. What I mean is that one of the major sources of tension is around your right kidney." I confirmed this for her by gently poking her right side.

"Yow, that hurts! But doesn't everyone hurt there?" She asked.

I then proceeded to poke her left side. There was no tenderness, and she nodded her head in understanding.

"Why did that hurt so much?" She asked. "I don't remember that being painful before."

"Primary restrictions are painful when you first get an injury. But, because they become relatively rigid, they tend not to be strained as easily, and so they become sources of *constant* irritation. Your brain is much more sensitive to changes in information, so a constant source of pain will sort of fade into the background. Other areas that now have to move abnormally because of the primary restriction can become more easily strained, and this is constantly changing depending on how you move. Therefore, your brain is more likely to register as painful those areas that are actually only compensating for the primary restrictions."

"I think I understand, but, it sure hurt when you poked it." she said rubbing her side. "It still hurts!"

"When I poked it," I continued, "I stimulated the primary restriction a little above the background level that your brain has gotten used to, and you were able to feel the pain that was really already there. It's only that you are now consciously aware of it again."

"But why would the kidney be injured in the first place?" She looked a little puzzled.

"That's a good question. I don't know how much you know about physics, but the denser a structure is, the more force of an impact it will absorb. This is why hitting a piece of wood makes a loud noise, while hitting a pillow does not make much sound." I demonstrated by knocking my knuckles against my desk and then on a cushion. "The denser material of the wood in the desk has lots of molecules packed closely together. When I bang on it with my knuckles, the molecules vibrate, and the molecules are set into vibration and easily bump into each other. The noise you hear is simply the mechanical energy I put into the wood being converted into sound energy. Material that is less dense will simply absorb a little of the energy, but most of it will pass right through without much effect since there are fewer molecules to collide with each other. So when I bang on the pillow, it doesn't make any sound.

"That's why, when you fall or are in a car accident, the force of the impact is absorbed more by the denser structures in your body." I explained. "So, can you tell me what is the densest substance in your body?"

"Well, I don't know." She responded. "Is it bone?"

"That's close." I answered. "Actually, it's water."

Her eyebrows raised in surprise at this. "Water!"

"Yes. You see, the molecules in water are as closely packed as they can be. That's why water is so heavy and is referred to as a noncompressible substance. This means you can't push the molecules in water any closer than they already are. So, when it is in an area where it can't spread out very easily, like in a container—think of the heart, the kidneys, the liver, the spleen, and even the head—it makes them act like big water balloons. Have you ever dropped a water balloon onto the pavement?" I asked.

She indicated with a smile that she had, and demonstrated with her hands, "Splat!"

"That's right!" I said. "In the same way, the water molecules inside these organs have only one way they can move when they absorb energy from an impact. They can only go outward. So the entire organ suddenly expands when the body experiences an injury like a fall or a car accident. That's why you may have heard about people who had a ruptured spleen after a car accident. That was because the spleen goes through periods during the day when it is full of blood (which is mostly water) and when it is almost empty. If it happens to be full when you have a serious impact like a car accident, then—kaboom! It explodes. That's because the spleen has a relatively thin wall around it. The other organs I mentioned are more protected, so they expand but they don't often explode. It's been said that in a car accident, there are actually three collisions: the cars with each other, the people inside the cars, and the organs inside the people. We find that the organs are usually involved, to some degree, in any form of impact injury."

I then demonstrated the effect of an impact to a water-filled internal organ using a Hoberman sphere (see figure 2-2 below).

"The tissues—muscle and fibrous tissue—around these organs are made of tensegrity material, like everything else in the body. When the water molecules inside them suddenly expand, the organ itself is forced outward. If the force is sufficient, the molecules can get stuck in the expanded, rigid position.

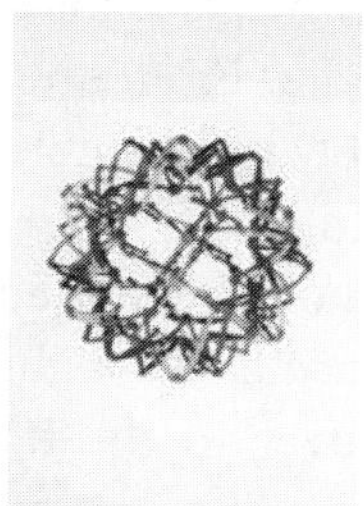

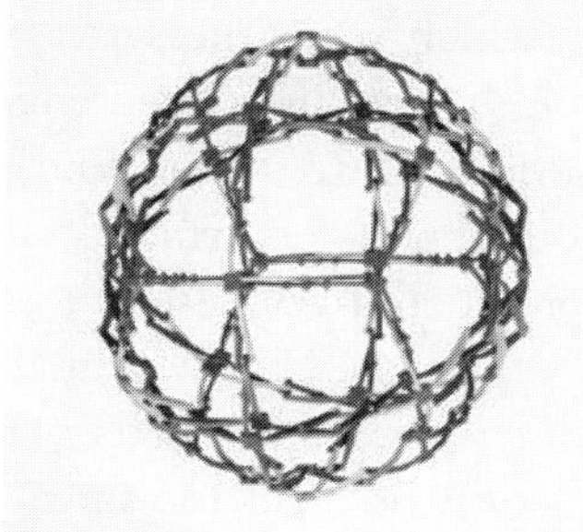

Figure 2-2: Collapsed and expanded Hoberman sphere

Since the tensegrity structure of the molecules is interconnected, the tightened and enlarged organs will pull the whole structure of the body out of alignment."

"That's interesting," said Sarah. "So, the water-filled organs absorb impact more easily because water is so dense, and when the organs get stuck and enlarged, they pull the rest of the body out of alignment. Is that right?"

"That's it exactly." I then pointed out an illustration of the body showing the location of the fluid-filled organs.

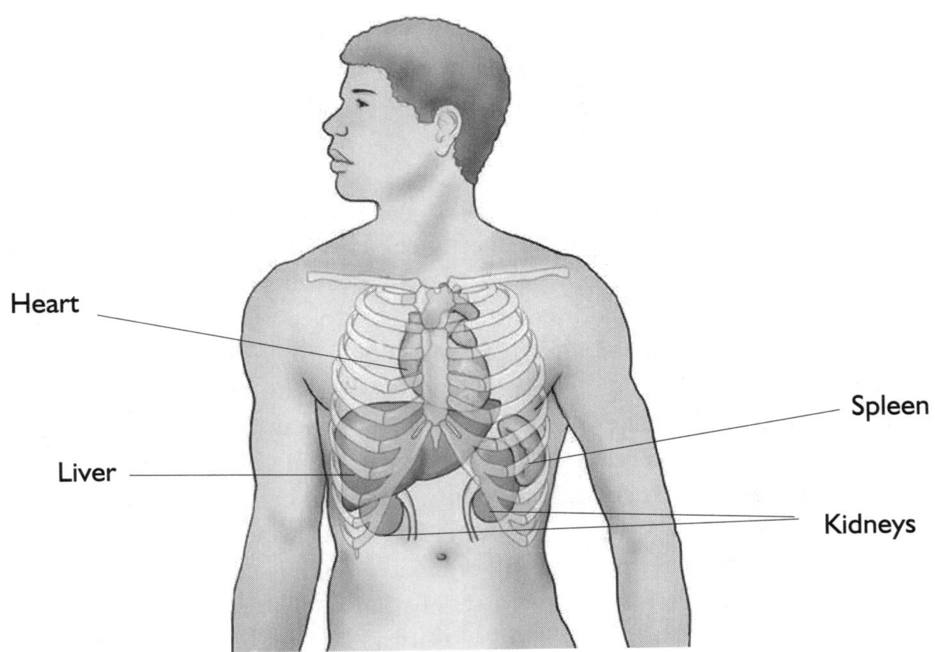

Figure 2-3: Fluid-filled organs

A PAIN IN THE NECK (OR BACK)

"But, why does my back hurt?" she asked. "I don't really feel pain in my kidneys."

"A lot of people ask that question," I continued, "and a lot of people have been trying to figure out why pain in the spine is such a common problem. You see, the spine is really important to our survival. It houses the spinal cord, which sends messages to the whole body and controls a lot of functions. If it is damaged, your life would be seriously threatened and you would likely die. From an evolutionary standpoint, it's even more serious. If we damage our spines, we would probably not be able to reproduce, and the species, especially our genetic contribution to it, would be threatened.

"So, nature has provided a very useful system to help us know when our spine, or any part of the body for that matter, is at risk. This system is pain. For example, you have a tight place—a primary restriction—around your right kidney. It is constantly pulling things over to the right, including your spine. So, if you try to turn or bend too far in certain directions, your spine can no longer go in that direction easily. This is not because there is a problem in the spine itself, but because the matrix connects everything in the body, including the tissues around your kidneys, to the muscles and ligaments around your spine. Since the joints in the spine are therefore not be able to move in a normal way, if you tried to force it to move in a certain direction, you might damage the spinal cord. Your body wants to prevent that, so it lets you know not to go too far in those directions by giving you a little reminder called pain."

"So," she inquired, "my spine is not the cause of the pain. It's only being strained by the problem around my kidney. But why does it hurt so much?"

"Nature wants to make sure that vital tissues like the spinal cord are protected, so we have a lot more pain nerve endings around our spine compared to other areas of the body. And this is why so many therapies have been developed to treat the spine—poking, prodding, cracking, stretching, cutting, adding hardware—all kinds of wild things. Most of them fail, in my opinion, because they're often looking in the wrong place. That doesn't mean that the problem can't be located right in the spine itself. It's just that it's a lot less common than people think."

THE HIP BONE'S CONNECTED TO . . . EVERYTHING!

"So, are most problems from injuries located in the organs?" she asked.

"Many are. When you guessed that bone is a very dense substance, you were right. It is the second-densest substance in the body because of the minerals deposited around its fibrous framework. It's actually a lot like reinforced concrete," I added.

"My chiropractor used to treat my bones, but the problem kept coming back." She stated.

"She wasn't really treating your bones. She was using your bones as levers to release restrictions in the joints around them. What I'm talking about is a strain right inside the bone itself. Most people think bone is rigid and hard, and that's just not true. Living, healthy bone is actually quite plastic and flexible. Let me show you."

She nodded agreement as I placed my hand on one thigh and then the other. I put some pressure on the middle of her left thighbone and pushed it toward the table. There was a feeling of suppleness of the muscle, and the bone itself had a small amount of give. When I did the same thing with the right thigh, the feeling was dramatically different. The thighbone felt like a piece of stone.

"Wow, I never knew there was such as difference. I could really feel that!" She exclaimed.

"I find that many problems are centered in the bones. Humans, because of our high center of gravity, are particularly prone to falling and landing on bones, like the hips and tailbone, or onto our knees, elbows, or shoulders. When the energy of the impact is absorbed into the bone they become rigid and often change their shape." I showed her the skeleton I keep in my office and pointed out some of the common bones that become injured with falls and strains.

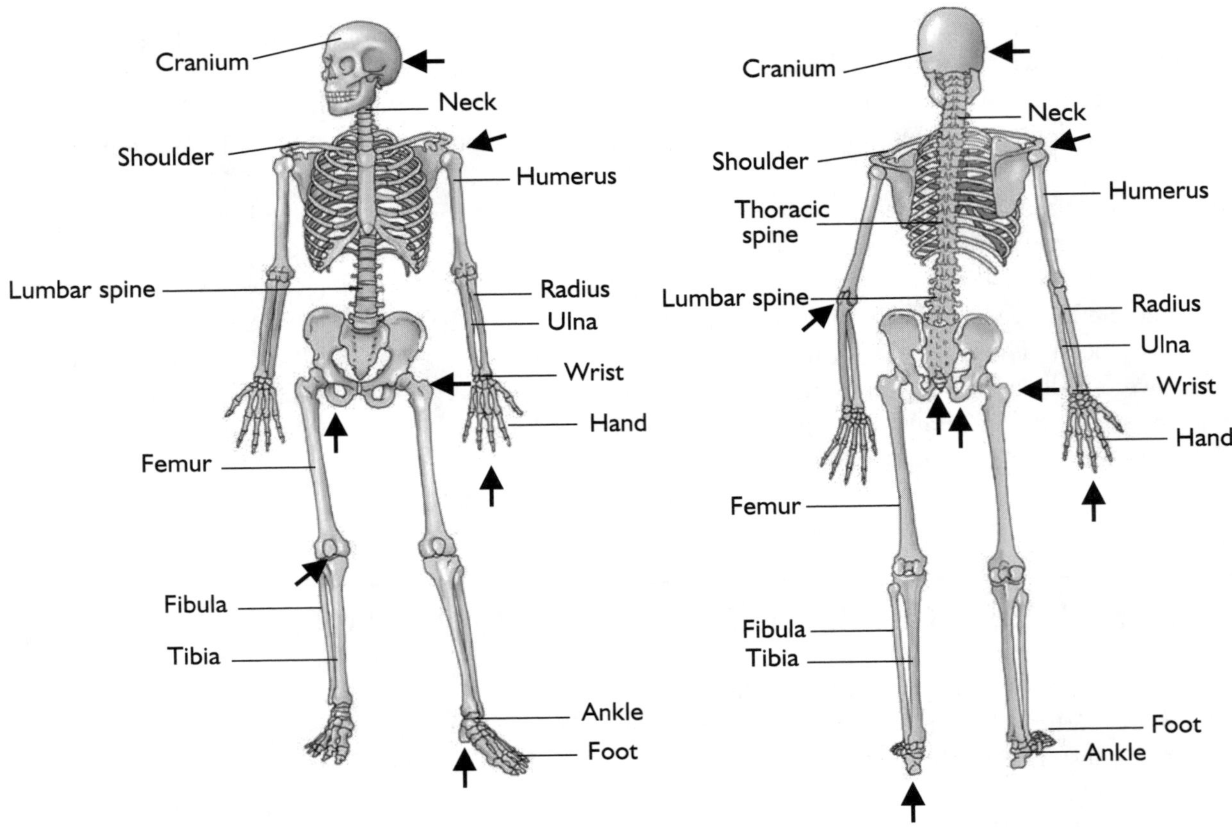

Figure 2-4: Skeleton showing common areas of strain and impact

Bone, like all tissues of the body, is part of the tensegrity matrix. It is composed of a fibrous framework embedded in a dense, crystalline, mineral matrix. The minerals in bone give it its hardness. This material, second only to water in density in the human body, also has the effect of concentrating the force of injury within bone as shown in figure 2-5, above. The belief that bone is a rigid, brittle substance is based on experience with dead (embalmed, dried, or cooked) material. Living bone, composed of the same tensegrity structure as every other part of the body, is actually slightly elastic and can flex, bend, twist, compress, and elongate to a certain degree in response to the normal forces of daily activities (Duncan 1995). It actually requires a significant amount of force to cause bone to fracture. In many cases, fractures occur in bones that have already undergone abnormal molecular changes rendering them less elastic and more brittle. When we fall onto our bottom or onto our knee or shoulder, we really feel it! The force entering the bones when they impact onto something else hard, like the floor or the ground, is significant. The molecules inside the bone absorb a lot of this energy, which may cause them to shift to the rigid, strained tensegrity structure. On impact, bones and the tissues around them appear to compress in line with the force entering them, and spread outward perpendicular to these forces. Think of dropping a lump of modeling clay onto a table. The lump will shorten from top to bottom and widen from side-to-side—the pancake effect. Bone may also be stretched, bent, or twisted in what we might call a straining injury. This can occur when you grab onto something with your hand as you fall. The bones (and joints) of the arm appear to become locked in a stretched state. Another common mishap is a twisting injury of the ankle. This may result in bending of the bones of the lower leg, as well as a strain within the ankle and foot joints.

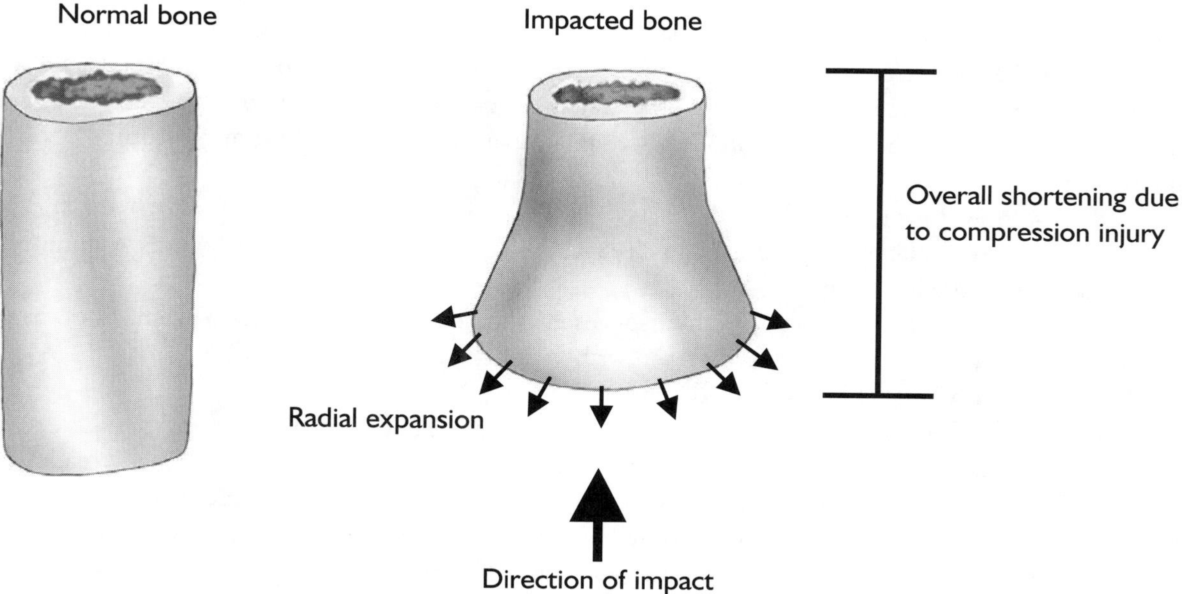

Figure 2-5: Effect of impact on bone

DISCOVERING OUR OWN POWER: HEALING OURSELVES

"So, what do you think Sarah? Does all of this make sense to you?" I asked.

"Well, yes. I guess so," she nodded while processing everything I had shown her. "It makes sense, and I could sure feel the softening when you put your hand over my ribs. And I really could feel that one of my thighbones was softer than the other. It's kind of amazing and sort of mysterious."

"Well it is amazing," I agreed, "but believe or not, it is something you can do for yourself as well."

"Who me? But I'm not a doctor." She protested. "I'm not a healer like you."

"Let me show you," I stated.

With that, I asked her to stand and bend forward. As expected, she experienced significant pain in her low back and, as a result, could only bend a few degrees. I then had her press down on one of her thighs to test the amount of tension in the muscle. She nodded that she could feel it. I then had her place her other hand on her right side, over her kidney area. I asked her to check the tension in her thigh again, and she was surprised to notice how it had softened. I had her take her hand away from her side and check her thigh muscle again. She noticed how it tightened again.

"Wow! I could really feel that," she exclaimed.

"Good," I said. "That was the same process that I used when I assessed you before. The area of the body you use to test another area is called the *indicator*. That simply means that it can indicate where the primary restriction is when you push on it. Your other hand is used to scan your whole body, and when you locate a primary restriction, the electrical field in your hand will shift the molecules toward the relaxed state. And since the matrix connects every part of the body to every other part, your whole body will relax just a little, which is why you feel your thigh muscle relax."

She nodded her understanding.

"Now place your hand over your right side again and leave it there for a few minutes. I just need to check on another patient." I showed her how to place her hand and relax back in the chair so she wouldn't get strained. I had her place her other hand on her thigh muscle and suggested she keep her hand on her side until she felt her thigh muscle relax even more. I then left and returned about five minutes later.

"Okay, so how do you feel?" I asked.

"Fine, I guess. Relaxed, maybe a little sleepy actually. You were right. After a few minutes, my thigh muscle relaxed a lot more."

"Great!" I said. "Now stand up." I then suggested she bend over at the waist again. She was quite surprised that she could bend much farther and with very little pain.

"Wow, did I do that?" She exclaimed.

"We all have the ability to help ourselves," I responded. "There's really not a mystery here. Matrix Repatterning is simply the direct application of our greater understanding of how the body really works. Even though your pain was in your back, you could see how your kidney was a more significant primary problem. Then, when you used your own normal electrical field to help shift it back toward normal, the muscles in your low back were able to relax and you were able move more easily and with less pain."

"That's amazing," she declared. "How can I learn more?"

"Just check at the front desk. We have regular self-treatment seminars where you can learn to provide yourself with basic treatments for many day-to-day strains and mishaps. It's sort of structural first aid."

"Sounds great. I'll definitely do that. So, where do we go from here?"

CLEARING OLD PATTERNS

"How about we go ahead and see if we can figure out what's going on in your body?" I suggested. She nodded enthusiastically. "Although you can help yourself with many minor injuries, my goal is to clear as many of the older injuries as possible, which may involve some more complex issues than you can address yourself."

"Makes sense to me." She agreed.

I proceeded to check her posture, the movement of each of her joints, the strength and tone of her muscles and the functioning of her nervous system. I showed her how I could read the pattern of tensions in her body. She was quite amazed how placing my hand over one area caused another area to relax, completely beyond her conscious control. She now understood that this process was a direct expression of the continuous molecular network of the body, the tensegrity matrix, which is the basis of Matrix Repatterning.

"While scanning your body with one of my hands," I explained, "I use my other hand to test the general state of tension. If I locate a primary molecular restriction with my scanning hand, you can feel how your rib cage relaxes when I press on it." I demonstrated this by first placing my scanning hand on her right knee. Her rib cage, which I was using as the indicator, immediately softened. "Placing my scanning hand over a normal area," I placed my scanning hand over her left knee, and the rib cage tightened again, "would have no effect on the overall level of tension in your body, since the two fields would be the same and no change would occur." She smiled, acknowledging her understanding. "This process of scanning and determining the precise location and nature of each of the primary restrictions within the body is, in fact, the basis of the Matrix Repatterning assessment."

I proceeded to examine her using this process. I documented my findings carefully and announced that I had been able to determine part of her injury pattern. This included compressed and bent bones (literally, bones that had become structurally distorted—not fractured—as a result of impact and strain injuries), as well as organs that had expanded as a result of these injuries.

I explained that the treatment process would be painless and gentle. In addition to what she had been able to do to correct the electrical field around her kidney, I would be applying some more precise pressure in different directions to effect a more complete resolution of the injury patterns. I warned her, however, that she might expect some aggravation of symptoms and possibly the surfacing of some old symptoms over the few days following treatment. She nonetheless agreed to allow me to proceed with treatment. This involved very gentle and precise pressure applied to the various parts of her body where I had located her primary restrictions.

"SHIFT" HAPPENS

"Your treatment was so gentle," she commented afterward. "I'm used to being pummeled, stretched, and cracked from head to toe. How can such a gentle treatment really do anything?"

"Let me show you something." I reached for an empty plastic water bottle. Then I held it up in front of her. "This bottle was molded into a specific shape. In other words, it has a built-in molecular memory that keeps it in this shape." She nodded.

"So," I continued, "if I apply a strong enough force, I can change its shape." I proceeded to smash the bottle with my other hand. The bottle was now collapsed in the middle and bent from top to bottom.

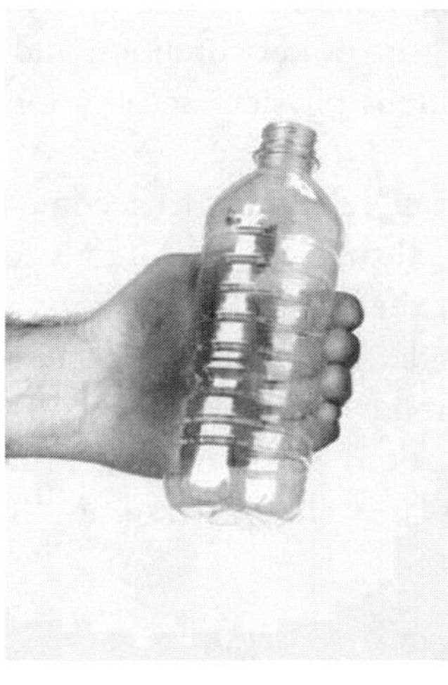

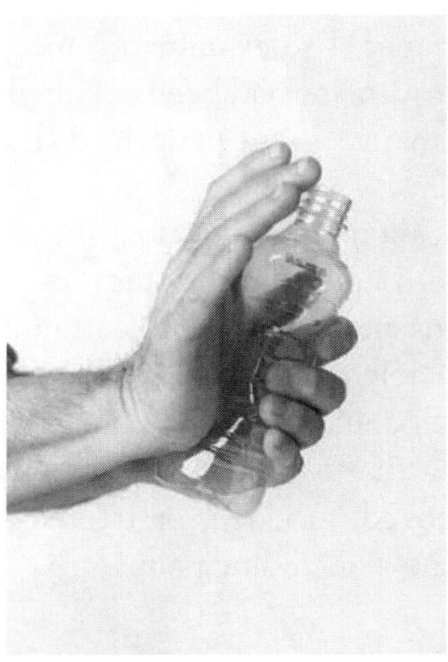

"You can see that it now has a new shape, which does not make it too useful as a bottle anymore. And you can see it took a lot of force to change its shape." Again, she agreed.

"Now, if you look closely, you can see that this shape change is greatest at certain specific locations." I pointed out the sharp folds where the plastic was most distorted from my blow. "If I can precisely locate these areas of greatest distortion and apply just the right amount of force . . ." I proceeded to apply gentle pressure to the folded areas on both sides of the flattened area. "Voila!" I said as the bottle instantly returned itself to its original shape.

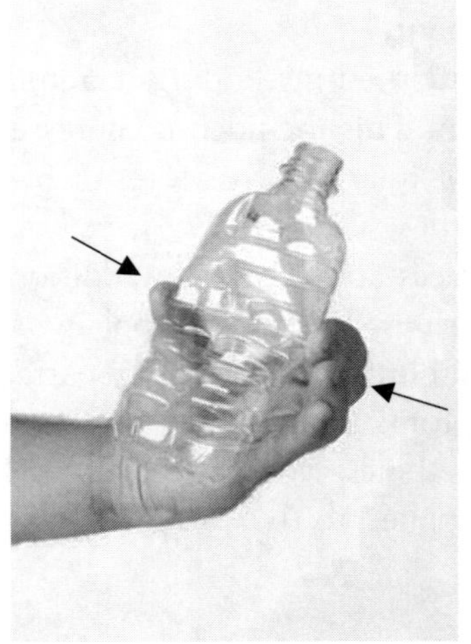

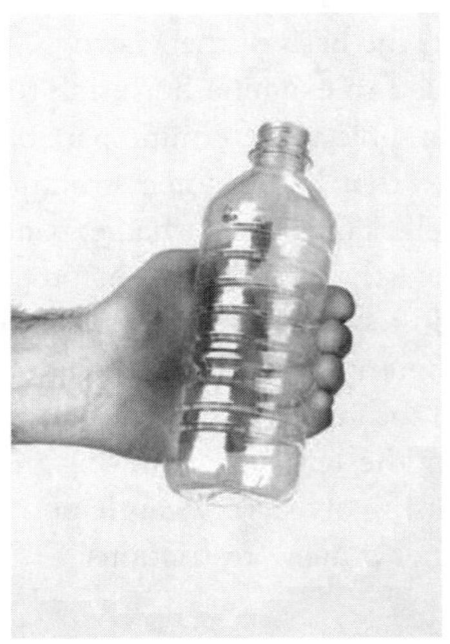

"You can see," I went on, holding up the restored vessel, "how little force was needed to restore its shape, compared to the force required to crush it initially. This is because the molecules in it were formed a certain way and this 'molecular memory' is retained, no matter how much it is distorted. Therefore, only minimal force—almost a gentle coaxing—is needed to release the original injury. Your body and the tensegrity matrix work the same way. Even though it may have taken a lot of force to create the problem, only minimal force or a normalizing electrical field, like you applied to your right kidney, is needed to correct it."

I proceeded to correct more of the tension patterns around her right kidney, the fibrous capsule around her liver, the pelvic bones and joints on the left, and her right femur (thighbone). Her range of motion improved immediately, and she reported that she had less pain with motion. After I completed the first treatment, I re-examined some of her restricted ranges of motion and was satisfied that some degree of improvement had been accomplished. Considering the nature of her condition and the amount of structural change I had performed, I suggested she avoid strenuous physical activity for a couple of days.

As our session drew to a close, I told her that her body had some relearning to accomplish, since its distorted pattern had been the status quo for a long time. I explained that the brain tends to get used to certain patterns and will adapt to certain levels of pain. This is why there is usually pain for a few days or weeks immediately after an injury and then the pain seems to subside. The brain is much more aware of changes (which could represent potential threats to survival) and tends to provide less conscious awareness of an area that is producing a relatively constant level of irritation. However, when these areas are stimulated—poked, prodded, or treated—the brain perceives this as a change, resulting in a renewed level of awareness, including pain.

Subsequent visits indicated that the restrictions that had been treated did not reoccur. Sarah's Cesarean section had resulted in a significant amount of scar tissue, which I treated using several other supportive therapies, including suggestions for home treatment (see appendix 2). The spine was not one of her primary areas, so I never did have to treat it. Several other layers of injury were released during subsequent treatments, and Sarah was able to get on with her life.

Sarah attended one of our self-treatment workshops and was able to help herself and her children with several minor injuries in the months following her treatment program. About six months later, she called to say she had fallen while skating and couldn't completely resolve one stubborn area. One treatment was all that was required to restore her body to optimal function.

CHAPTER 3

Pain Is Not the Problem

If we listen carefully, the message of pain can help us immeasurably. It is simply a message that something it out of balance. Matrix Repatterning can help us address the underlying structural causes of pain. When we correct the real problem, we will make an important discovery: that pain itself is not the problem.

PURPOSE OF PAIN

One of the greatest assets you can have in taking charge of your health is an understanding of your own body, the relationship between health and disease, and the factors governing each. The medical community has largely ignored the idea of the disease process and instead has relied on a huge arsenal of drugs and radical, invasive procedures to reduce symptoms. Ironically, symptoms are a crucial method of communication that the body relies upon to alert us to serious threats to our health. Symptoms can be compared to your neighbor telling you that your house is on fire. If you proceed to put a strip of tape over your neighbor's mouth, you have effectively dealt with this annoying symptom. The problem is, your house would probably burn down, and you would never know it until it was too late.

Symptoms, such as pain, are not the enemy. They provide valuable information that something is wrong and needs your attention. Honor the aches and pains as opportunities to receive important messages designed to direct your attention to conditions or areas that require some form of remedial action. Our society has largely been conditioned to fear pain and this only adds to our distress. As we begin to improve our understanding of the body and the true purpose of pain, we will have an opportunity to improve our health and our lives. Remember, the Chinese symbol for "crisis" is the same as the one for "opportunity."

THE MESSAGE OF PAIN

The tensegrity matrix forms the basis of a new understanding of the mechanics of the body and how it is affected by injury, literally at the molecular level. We mentioned earlier what happens when we break a bone. When the bone is first injured, it is extremely painful. This pain is a result of powerful stimulation of the pain nerve endings (receptors) due to the strain or overstretching of the tissues around the area, along with inflammation and local swelling. Once a cast is applied and the inflammation begins to subside, the injured area, now unable to move or become strained, soon becomes symptom free. As we begin to move around and engage in normal activities however, other areas of the body must now move in abnormal ways to compensate for the restrictive effect of the cast. As a result, other areas often become strained and painful.

Similarly, a severe strain or impact may cause a local restriction to develop in the injured area, causing it to become relatively rigid compared to other parts of the body. This has the effect of limiting local movement and causing other parts of the body to compensate, in much the same way as having a cast in place.

The tensegrity matrix, linking each cell of the body to every other cell of the body, efficiently and consistently transmits tension from the primary restriction throughout the entire structure. Therefore, many other parts of the body are then forced to compensate for the tension patterns created by the primary restriction, leading to irritation and pain in these secondary areas. The area of primary restriction often becomes less painful over time if it is not forced to move excessively. However, it continues to be a source of background tension, causing many other parts of the body to have limited or abnormal motion.

The area of primary molecular restriction within the matrix is not easily strained by most activities, since it is now in a relative state of restriction (similar to wearing a cast for a broken bone). Therefore, under most circumstances, it serves no adaptive purpose for the brain to continue to perceive this area as painful. It is often only when the primary area of restriction is stimulated by, for example, direct pressure or excessive strain, that it again becomes painful. Please note that the area of the primary restriction continues to be an area of irritation. This is why it is always tender to the touch or pressure. This is due to the fact that the brain tends to adapt to a constant level of stimulation. We'll discuss this phenomenon further below.

For example, a primary restriction in the pelvis may lead to an abnormal pattern of movement in, say, the shoulder. The shoulder will be forced to move abnormally in certain directions to compensate for the parts that are being held rigid by the primary source of restriction. The ligaments around a joint, like the shoulder, are richly supplied with pain receptors (specialized nerve endings). These tissues may become overstretched and damaged. Chemicals, such as histamine, are released by the damaged cells and create a chain reaction of cellular response referred to as *inflammation*. These chemicals stimulate the pain receptors, which in turn produce nerve impulses that are transmitted to pain centers in the brain.

The resulting pain would then be felt in the shoulder, which is actually being strained due to the tension coming from a source of restriction in the pelvis. Conventional treatment directed at the inflamed shoulder would provide only temporary relief, since the primary source of the problem had not been addressed. Certain movements of the arm would tend to engage the tension pattern coming from the pelvis, and the pain in the shoulder would re-emerge. People usually adapt to these limitations and eventually learn to avoid moving certain ways to avoid triggering their pain, but as soon as they do too much, the pain comes right back.

THE DECISION TO FEEL PAIN

The brain is continuously comparing information from incoming nerve pathways. The brain also filters out a great deal of the incoming impulses. Indeed, if we were consciously aware of all of the pain signals from all of the different areas throughout the body, we would be in a practically catatonic state, completely overloaded and unable to function. Thus the brain is constantly adapting and allowing only those stimuli that are above a certain threshold to rise to the conscious level (Wall 2000). This is also why the painful areas appear to be constantly shifting and changing. Depending on our activities or other variables, such as body chemistry or stress factors, one area may become a more predominant source of nerve stimulation compared to another area.

The more acute the pain or the more critical the area of the body involved (areas usually supplied with a higher concentration of pain receptors), the higher the priority it is for the brain to bring it to our conscious awareness. This determines the *awareness threshold*, below which a source of information such as a pain signal will essentially remain invisible to the conscious brain. Symptoms like pain are important only because they provide feedback to the sufferer that certain activities may produce strain beyond the level of tolerance of the structures involved. This can protect the area from becoming seriously damaged.

No one wins when the focus of treatment is solely on pain. The underlying problem may still be lurking and slowly undermining health, while the pain itself may be located in a completely different area. Pain will usually be present within the local area of primary strain or impact right after an injury occurs. This is due to the initial mechanical distortion of the muscles, ligaments, or bones as well as the trauma to internal structures such as organs. This results in local inflammation, including swelling and increased blood flow. This usually lasts for a brief period—two to three weeks at most. After this acute phase of the injury, the nervous system generally adapts to the new status quo within the tissues and the threshold for allowing pain symptoms to rise to the conscious level is raised.

A source of irritation (such as a physical injury along with the molecular changes associated with it) that has been in place for a period of time, and which is not being continually aggravated, tends to be considered by the brain as nonthreatening. This level of irritation becomes the new threshold and eventually drops below the conscious level of awareness. It is only if these areas are re-injured or excessively stressed that they rise to the level of conscious perception and are again reported as pain.

This is how nature allows us to continue functioning without the hindrance of unpleasant and stress-inducing symptoms, such as pain. The organism is free to pursue the all-important tasks of survival, such as feeding and procreation, without the distraction of a constant barrage of symptoms that serve no useful purpose. Certain people experience chronic pain due to a chemical or neurological imbalance that prevents this filtering mechanism from functioning effectively. This has been identified as one of the mechanisms in a condition called fibromyalgia (see chapter 6).

Symptoms such as pain are a subjective expression of objective information. The brain interprets data arising from sensory receptors in various tissues and determines, through comparison with many other sources of information, its relative significance. The *pain threshold*, determines the level at which a source of irritation will become a conscious awareness of pain. The criteria for determining whether any particular set of incoming nerve impulses will be interpreted as pain are a complex set of variables. These variables include the strength and location of the stimulus, the background state of the nervous system, chemical and hormonal influences, and the emotional state of the individual, among others.

These factors tend to exert an influence on the threshold mechanism located in the brain. In a sense, the brain keeps score and awards the source of irritation with the most points (the greatest number of certain types of nerve impulses) the prize of rising to the conscious level as pain. The awareness of pain could be considered as sort of a popularity contest.

LOCATION, LOCATION, LOCATION

The location of the source of pain is an important factor in determining its potential to rise to the level of conscious awareness. For example, head pain and back pain are extremely common. It is well-known that the fibrous coverings of the spinal cord and the brain, called *meninges*, contain a high concentration of pain nerve endings (Wall 2000). These areas could be considered prime locations in terms of relevance to our survival. Loss of the ability to move, feel sensations, and make decisions would substantially undermine our chances of survival. Therefore, if the nervous system were threatened by direct injury due to pressure on the spinal cord or the spinal nerves, there would be an advantage if there were a feedback system to prevent excessive movement in certain directions that could damage any of these structures. Pain serves this role very well. You feel the pain, and you become more careful in your movement.

This may be why back and neck pain are so common and have been the subject of so much medical attention and intervention. The location of the pain, however, says nothing of the mechanical origin of the imbalance that led to the spinal disturbance. This may be why so many of the measures developed to treat these areas have been less than effective.

MIND-BODY RELATIONSHIPS

How each of us perceives pain is also determined by attitudes and beliefs about pain. Studies also show that people with a positive outlook on life tend to feel pain less intensely. There is scientific evidence that our attitude affects our biochemistry, including the relative amounts of pain-producing and pain-relieving chemicals (Dienstfrey 1991; Pert 1997). Once we understand this relationship, it is quite possible that refocusing our thinking will aid our ability to counteract the debilitating effects of pain.

One of the goals of this book is to demystify the way our bodies work and to dispel many of the myths associated with pain. Matrix Repatterning offers a specific method for locating the source of structural imbalance and resolving many of the issues producing pain. This can go a long way to reducing the distress and fear that often accompany pain.

Many people have found that simple distraction, like getting busy with a hobby or other enjoyable activity, can often help reduce the intensity of pain signals. Other practices like meditation or creative visualization may also be of benefit.

TREATMENT AT THE SOURCE

Pain appears to be a relatively nonspecific and unreliable indicator of the actual source of an imbalance in the body. This is why symptoms such as pain can seem to move around and come and go under mysterious circumstances. As a result, diagnosis and treatment based on symptoms like pain are often frustrating and fruitless, since they apply only to the secondary effects and not the primary condition behind those symptoms.

Typically, an individual attempts to alleviate the painful messages from an injury or strain by seeking relief through medication or some form of therapeutic intervention. Painkillers may succeed in nullifying the painful impulses. Conventional therapy is usually directed to the area of complaint and might include electrotherapy, exercise, manipulation, injections, or if the condition is sufficiently progressed, surgery. Some of these techniques may produce a reduction in symptoms—for a while—until the person re-strains that or some other area, and more pain signals are produced.

Since the primary source of the problem is rarely addressed, the abnormal mechanical stresses on joints and surrounding structures continue to develop. The joints that have to compensate for a restriction elsewhere in the body are only able to move in certain ways because other directions are limited. This creates an imbalance in joint movement, therefore accelerating wear and tear on these tissues.

If you listen carefully, the message of pain can help you immeasurably. It is simply a message that something is out of balance. Matrix Repatterning can help you address the underlying structural causes of pain. The goal of Matrix Repatterning is to identify the source of the tension patterns that may be causing mechanical strain and abnormal function, which lead to pain. Treatment is always directed to these areas, despite the actual location of the pain.

DEALING WITH PAIN

Once pain has been established for a long period of time, there are nerve pathways that can become hypersensitive to this form of information. These pathways may develop a pattern of response that lead to the perception of significant pain with even a small amount of stimulation. This is referred to as a *facilitated pathway* (Denslow, Korr, and Krems 1947). This response may persist even when many of the structural or mechanical issues are improved. An analogy of this phenomenon is a person being punched in the arm all day long. Then another person comes along and strokes the same area with a feather. "Ouch! That hurts! Darn feather!" might be the response. In fact, the arm has been irritated and the pain receptors and nerves connecting them to them brain have been hypersensitized. The feather is a much smaller stimulus, but due to the hypersensitivity of the pathway, the response is heightened such that the pain is out of proportion to the current situation.

At the cellular level, the actual mechanism of stimulation of the nervous system's pain receptors is the release of chemicals by cells as part of the inflammatory process. Inflammation is the body's response to irritation from any source. This could be a splinter, an infection, or damaged cells resulting from a severe strain or blow. It involves a number of chemical responses whose overall purpose is to protect the body from the most serious of all threats—the spread of infection. The body does not differentiate, however, between a closed injury (no break in the skin) and an open one. An open injury involves the potential for infection, while a strain is a closed injury where this threat is not present. Unfortunately, the inflammatory response is the same in either case, and in the case of a closed injury it can produce a number of unpleasant side effects. This is because blood and other fluids tend to accumulate in the area of injury without an actual break in the skin. This accumulation causes significant swelling and pressure on pain-sensitive structures.

Therefore it is essential that we have strategies to overcome the negative effects of inflammation and the pain associated with it once they have served their protective roles in preventing further injury. Simple measures such as ice (or *cryotherapy*) have been used successfully for centuries. Cold counteracts the increased swelling associated with the inflammation. Cold helps to constrict blood and lymph vessels, which have dilated, allowing fluid to accumulate in the area. For more information on the use of ice therapy to counteract the effects inflammation, please refer to "Cold Therapy" in appendix 2.

There are several methods of dealing with the facilitated or hypersensitive pain pathways. There are numerous pain medications, available over-the-counter or by prescription, which can alter the perception of pain for a period of time. These medications, along with muscle-relaxing drugs or herbal equivalents can help to break the pain-muscle spasm cycle. Reactive muscle spasm may contribute to the severity of the pain by reducing local blood flow and thereby accentuating the accumulation of inflammatory tissue fluids and the pain they produce. This temporary relief can often be sufficient to break the cycle of pain and allow the level of discomfort to be restored to a more tolerable level. This respite can have beneficial effects both physically and psychologically. Long term use of pain medications, however, is not advised, since this can lead to dependency and allow the ongoing mechanical issues to persist unchecked. Remember, pain does serve a useful purpose, as it limits certain activities, which might lead to damage of joints or other tissues. The short-term use of pain medications may be beneficial as long as other measures are instituted to overcome the underlying causes of pain.

MENTAL ALIGNMENT

As I touched on earlier, mounting evidence supports the connection between the body and the mind. The tensegrity matrix may explain part of this important level of communication. The way the nervous system communicates with the body could be compared to phone lines that connect one part of the brain to a specific part of the body (Oschman 2000). This is a very fast and defined pathway of transmitting information between these areas. The matrix, on the other hand, could be compared with the Internet. The Internet communicates in a more general way, finding the pathway(s) of least resistance through several possible transmission routes within a large grid. Because of the electronic and structural properties of the matrix, conscious or unconscious thoughts (electrical signals) may be translated by different tissues throughout the body in different ways. For example, worry or fear could be translated as increased muscle tension in the shoulders, increased adrenaline production in the adrenal glands, stimulation of the sweat glands, and increased heart rate and rate of breathing. Most of these responses are automatic and unconscious. They all serve the overall purpose of meeting a perceived threat, which mental stress simulates even though no physical threat may actually exist at the time.

Extreme or persistent pain may be perceived by the body as a form of threat. It may begin to dominate our thoughts and our entire life experience. Additionally, the pain may be associated with other negative thoughts or beliefs. For example, you may have been told various things about why you have the pain. You may have been given a "diagnosis" that could have caused you some worry about the state of your health and especially the condition of the area in which the pain is felt. Then, every time you feel even a small amount of pain, it can trigger an emotional response of worry or fear, which in turn increases your awareness of the area. All of these negative associations serve to magnify the degree to which the pain is perceived (Wall 2000).

As we've seen, pain serves a very useful purpose. It prevents us from further injuring ourselves or damaging tissues. Unfortunately, when the pain is located in a secondary area that is compensating for a primary restriction in another location, it can be deceptive as to the actual source of the problem. The key to resolving the cause of the pain is to restore optimal function. This means that the primary restrictions need to be located and successfully treated. Matrix Repatterning has the potential to address these issues directly and efficiently. Proper body mechanics can be restored, either by the self-treatment methods listed in chapter 5 or through professional intervention by a Matrix Repatterning practitioner.

Pain may continue after the body is functionally improved due to the residual effects within the nerve pathways to the pain centers of the brain (the facilitated pathway), as well as the psychological factors mentioned above. Therefore, even though the body is functionally improved, the pain may continue. The persisting pain itself then may become a source of stress, which can have detrimental effects on your health. Several studies document the effects of stress on the immune system, digestive tract, cardiovascular system, and many other systems of the body (Dienstfrey 1991).

Pain can produce a number of physical and psychological responses. One of the most common is muscle tension. Dr. John Sarno, in his landmark book *Mind Over Back Pain*, discusses the importance of muscle tension as a direct expression of the ongoing cycle of pain and its association with mental stress (1982). He found that by changing the individual's belief about their condition—defusing much of the unnecessary anxiety related to a real or imagined "diagnosis"—he was able to not only dispel many of these misconceptions, but also encourage a significant reduction in the muscle tension (which he termed Tension Myositis Syndrome) and its effects on maintaining the cycle of pain and debility. Muscle tension itself can lead to a local reduction in blood flow, causing cell damage and the resulting accumulation of the chemicals that encourage inflamation—and hence more pain (Hatfaludy, Hannsky, and Vandenburgh 1989). This can become a vicious cycle as the pain and increasing muscle tension escalate.

Mounting evidence supports the idea that psychological factors affect everything from heart function to digestion to the effectiveness of the immune system. When it comes to the issue of pain anywhere in the body, the mind can be recruited as an ally in the battle against the cycle of pain and inflammation. As mentioned above, Dr. Sarno has successfully educated individuals to help them better understand their condition. By overcoming their fear as to the underlying cause of persisting muscle tension, many have been able to resolve their pain issues.

There are various ways you can enlist the aid of your own mind to help you relieve pain and assist your body toward optimal function. First and foremost, it is essential that you dispel many of the misconceptions you may have been offered or read about in your search for answers related to your pain. Dr. Sarno discusses a direct link between our belief as to the cause of our pain and the perceived severity of our symptoms (1991). The reality of many of these diagnoses has come under suspicion. Studies have shown a significant disparity between the presumed condition and the actual findings at the time of surgery or on follow-up examination (Moseley et al. 2002). Unfortunately, to the untrained layperson, many of the these pronouncements, couched in dire terms and usually associated with a picture of continual decline and eventual disability, serve only to heighten fear and the ensuing spiral of increasing pain and distress.

Part of the purpose of this book is to dispel some of these myths. It is remarkable how a positive attitude coupled with the practical and safe methods outlined here can provide significant relief from pain while also restoring optimal health. We encourage you to take charge of your health with confidence in the healing powers of your own body.

A SIMPLE MENTAL EXERCISE TO HELP REDUCE PAIN

Pain has a way of getting our attention, sometimes more than we would like. The fact that we are paying attention to it, along with some of our own fears and misconceptions about why it may be present, tends to intensify the pain. The exercise outlined below is designed to alter your perception of pain by using a positive mental image to reduce its intensity and degree.

Pain may be defined by the area in which it is felt. As such, it may have a definite boundary. The size and sharpness of this boundary, as perceived by the mind, has an effect on how strongly you feel the pain. Your mind is capable of affecting this boundary through the power of visualization.

EXERCISE: DISSOLVING THE PAIN

1. Find a comfortable position, sitting or lying down.
2. Focus your attention on the area of pain.
3. Define the current boundary of the painful area. How large is it? What does it look like or feel like? (For example, what is its color? Is it sharp, knifelike, or heavy and dull? Is the outline thick or thin?
4. Visualize the boundary beginning to soften around the edges. Imagine it sort of melting or dissolving, eventually become relatively undefined. As you do this, focus on your breathing, making it comfortably full and relaxed.
5. Next, imagine the area of pain beginning to shrink away from the former outline. Do this in several steps, allowing the painful area to become smaller and smaller, each time feeling the new boundary softening as in the step above.

With a little practice, you should be able to diminish the intensity of your pain and therefore help reduce your overall level of stress and tension. This can help to break the cycle of pain-stress-pain that can often become so debilitating. Don't worry if you're not successful right away. You may find it necessary to apply some of the Matrix Repatterning techniques a few times before the pain begins to reduce enough for you to begin applying these visualization exercises. The combination of both the physical and mental approaches may be more powerful than either might be individually. Using some of these simple tools to help reduce the mental focus on pain, along with the gentle hands-on techniques you'll be learning in the rest of the book, can form a powerful team to get you back into a more joyful, pain-free existence more quickly.

CHAPTER 4

Matrix Repatterning Self-Assessment

In this chapter you will be given the tools to be able to locate the source of many of the structural imbalances that may have arisen due to strains and falls, sports injuries, minor motor vehicle collisions, and the effects of scar tissue. These sources of restriction may be the underlying cause of your susceptibility to many of the aches and pains you may be experiencing. You will be able to efficiently assess the areas of restriction and treat them using gentle, noninvasive methods. These techniques are safe for all members of the family and can help with many acute injuries, which happen with surprising frequency, especially with young, active children and those involved in sports.

THE ELUSIVE SOURCE

When you first get injured, the place you feel pain is the part that was directly affected. This could be the knee or hip you have fallen onto, the shoulder you strained while grabbing onto something as you unceremoniously tripped over a toy in the middle of the night, or your back after lifting something too heavy the wrong way. Pain is the feedback system that alerts you to the damaged part in order to prevent further injury. It encourages you to rest or to alter your activity in such a way as to avoid further straining the affected area.

As discussed in the preceding chapter, the brain is highly adaptive to pain signals. The area of the body that is irritated will send information to the conscious level of the brain in the form of pain or some other symptom. However, once the inflammation (the body's chemical and cellular reaction to damaged tissue) is stabilized (and if the area is not actively being stressed beyond its new, more limited, range of movement), the brain tends to accept the new condition of these tissues as the status quo. In other words, the area of primary injury will usually no longer be painful after a few days or within one to two weeks, under most conditions. But this doesn't mean the problem has gone away. It just means that your brain has adapted to it so you can get on with your life. As we now understand, the tensegrity matrix connects every part of the body to every other part. As a result, other parts of your body may begin to register distress, discomfort, or abnormal function as they are forced to move abnormally due to the primary problem.

The degree to which these compensations become a nuisance depends on how much and what types of physical activity you engage in. If you work sitting at a desk all day, you're less likely to aggravate the existing strain patterns—unless you decide to become a weekend warrior and exert yourself by participating in some vigorous sports activity or a major yard-work project. If you are active in athletics (including that future Olympic sport, housework), you may be pushing your body to the limit. As a result, you may be much more aware of the presence of imbalances, either due to some limitation in the performance of a certain activity or due to pain. You would therefore be much more likely to seek help at an earlier stage of imbalance due to this heightened awareness.

The purpose of treatment in the Matrix Repatterning Program is to restore the normal molecular pattern in parts of the body where injury has changed the tensegrity matrix to a rigid form. As you'll recall, these primary restrictions are the sources of tension that may result in painful conditions and other health problems. In many cases these areas are not painful themselves, but they are always tender to the touch. Primary restrictions also cause other parts of the body to move and function abnormally, resulting in strain and pain. They may also play an important role in creating abnormal function at the cellular level, which could lead to more serious health issues (Ingber 1998, 2002).

ZEROING IN ON THE PRIMARY RESTRICTION

The tensegrity matrix, as we have already discussed, forms one continuous fabric throughout the body. At the site of primary injury, the molecular structure becomes rigid. It becomes a source of tension that distorts the overall fabric and the mechanical function of the entire body. This causes strain and pain in other areas that now have to function within this disturbed pattern. Joints in other areas of the body attempting to move beyond certain limits will encounter resistance and an alteration of their normal pattern of movement. Joints, ligaments, and other fibrous tissues, which contain many pain nerve endings, will tend to become strained and irritated. Joints that have to move in an abnormal way due to the strain patterns imposed on them may also become subject to wear and tear.

The primary restriction is always in a state of irritation and inflammation. Any subjective decrease in the sensation of pain is because the brain has adapted to the constant level of stimulation. When the area of the primary restriction is stimulated, as by poking or prodding with your fingers, you effectively increase the signals going to your brain, and you will find that the area is actually very tender. This may surprise you, since the area may not have been noticeably painful for some time since the original injury. This tenderness is a useful clue that you have found the correct area to treat. *Pain* could be defined as a feeling of discomfort in the body, while *tenderness* is discomfort produced by direct stimulation (poking). In fact, the area where you may have been feeling pain is usually not as tender to the touch as the primary area, since it is often only compensating for the main area of restriction.

The goal, in terms of truly restoring ideal health and function to the matrix, is to apply the appropriate therapy to the appropriate area. We know that pain may or may not be present in the primary site due to the adaptive nature of the brain. The Matrix Repatterning Self-Assessment is designed to help you discover for yourself the primary sources of tension within your body, and thus to be able to apply a corrective procedure to treat the source of the problem—not just the symptoms.

WHAT YOU'RE GOING TO LEARN

The purpose of the Matrix Repatterning Program is to provide the average person, who is not trained as a health-care provider, with the means to self-assess and treat minor day-to-day and certain chronic (long-term) conditions. This could be considered a structural first-aid program, helping you alleviate many of the strains and other injuries you may encounter in your active life. Matrix Repatterning Self-Assessment consists of hte following components:

- A systematic method for determining whether you have a structural imbalance (Body Check).
- A simple method for locating primary restrictions (Body Scan).

IMPROVING SENSITIVITY

To begin, try this sensitivity-training exercise. This can help you understand the very real nature of the tensegrity matrix, and how it can be such an important influence on your body. With these exercises, you will be tensing one area of the body and feeling the effects in another. This mimics the effect of a primary restriction. At first you may find it difficult to feel these sensations. Don't worry. As you begin to achieve a greater degree of balance in your body through the Matrix Repatterning Program, you may be able to feel these subtle changes more easily.

EXERCISE: SENSITIVITY TRAINING

1. Sit up straight in a chair.
2. Try to be aware of the amount of tension in your neck and shoulders.
3. Curl the toes of one foot under and then point your toes up toward your head. Repeat this several times, being aware of the feeling in your neck area. What you may feel is a slight tightening of some of the muscles in your neck as you curl your toes in one direction and other muscles, usually on the opposite side of your neck, as you curl them in the opposite direction.
4. Next, extend one arm out to the side and slightly behind you (do not overstretch). Stretch out your hand and extend the fingers backward. Try to be aware of the feeling in your neck and shoulder area. You may notice a slight change in the degree of tension in your neck and shoulders.

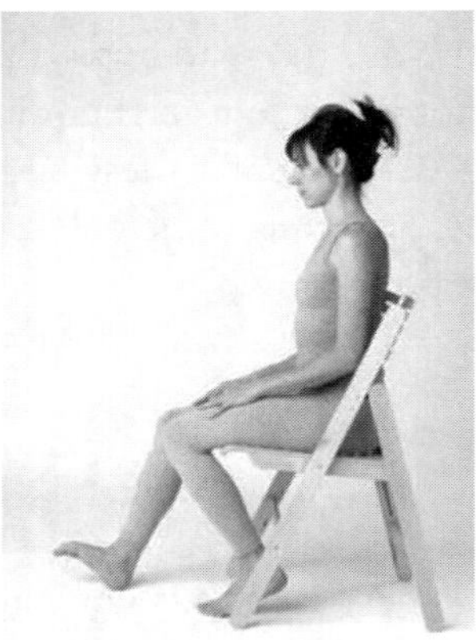

Toe curl, down: Curl the toes down toward the floor. Notice the sensation of tension in the neck and shoulders.

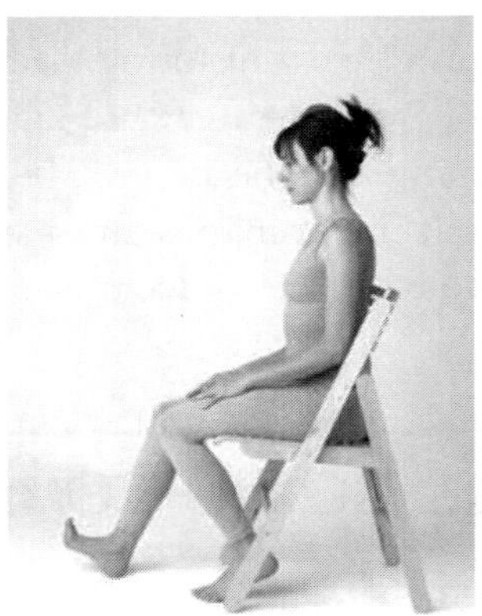

Toe curl, up: Curl the toes up toward your head. Notice the sensation of tension in the neck and shoulders.

5. Resting your arm on your thigh, curl your fingers in toward the palm of your hand and make a fist. You may notice an increase in tension in your neck and shoulders as you do this.

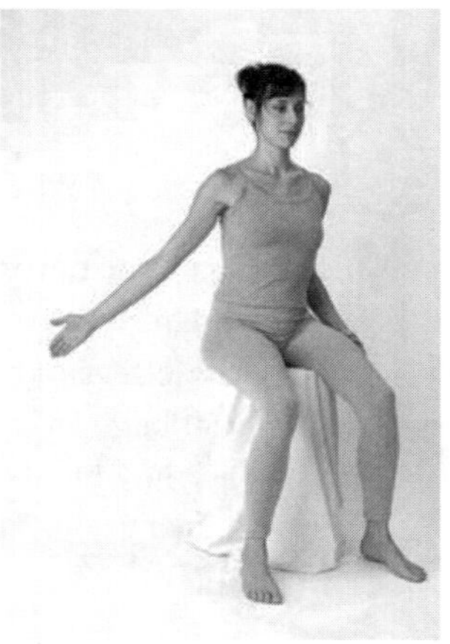

Finger extension: Extend your arm behind you and extend your fingers. Notice the sensation of tension in the neck and shoulders.

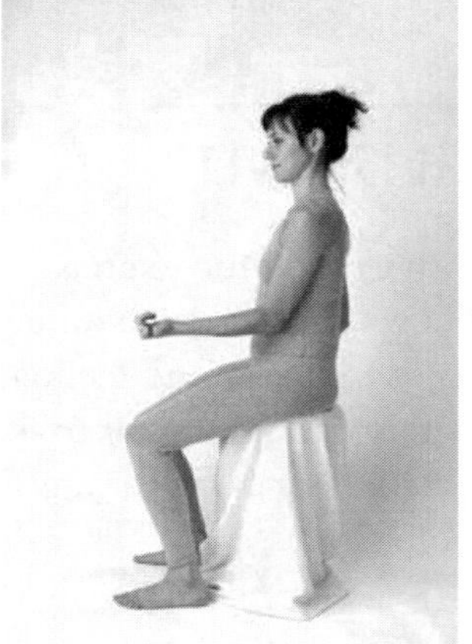

Finger flexion: With your arm held at your side, curl the fingers toward the palm of the hand to make a fist. Notice the sensation of tension in the neck and shoulders.

Once you have performed some of the self-treatment methods outlined below, try the sensitivity test again. You may find that you are now more sensitive to these subtle changes in your body.

The effect of moving one part of the body and feeling a change in tension in another part can only be explained by the continuous connection between every part of the body created by the tensegrity matrix. Since every part of the body is made of the same stuff (the tensegrity matrix), every part of the body behaves in the same manner as every other part at the molecular level. Movement, circulation, nerve function, digestion, hormone and enzyme production, even genetic expression (how our chromosomes function) appear to be determined by the state of balance within the tensegrity matrix.

SELF-ASSESSMENT

The self-assessment process involves two steps. The first step, the Body Check, is to determine whether or not you have a structural imbalance. The second step, the Body Scan, is to actually locate the primary restrictions, which are the sources of the imbalance.

Step 1: Body Check

Before you perform any specific tests of the body, it may be useful to determine what, if any, are its current limitations. To do this, you can perform some objective tests and make a note of any abnormal findings. We refer to these tests as a Body Check. This check will help to confirm the reality of your results, since pain by itself is not a very reliable indication of success. The Body Check is a useful guide to help you determine the need for possible structural therapy and to confirm the changes (range of motion, flexibility, muscle balance, strength, etc.) accomplished with your treatment. Make a note of each of the tests below that seems to indicate an imbalance and then recheck them after you have completed your treatment. Also, please remember to move within your comfort level during all of these procedures. Never force any of the movements.

You may choose to perform this process only one time as a means of obtaining a perspective on the general state of your body. You may wish to use it as a way of checking your state of balance before each treatment or simply from time to time as a preventive measure. If you have an acute injury, such as a blow to a part of your body, an impact, or a significant strain, you may simply check that area using the assessment process and treat it using the electrical or the mechanical treatments as described later. In other words, there is no need to check the entire body each time, unless you have ongoing pain of unknown origin or pain that comes on with only mild to moderate activity.

Posture

1. Stand facing a full-length mirror either nude or wearing tights or underwear.

2. Notice the position of your head. Are your ears and eyes parallel with the ground? Are they tilted? Is your head rotated in one direction or the other or tilted to one side?

3. Check the level of your shoulders. Does one of your hands reach farther down your thigh than the other? Are your shoulders positioned forward on one side or the other?

4. Notice the position of your hips. Do they seem pulled over to one side or the other? Do they appear to be rotated forward or backward?

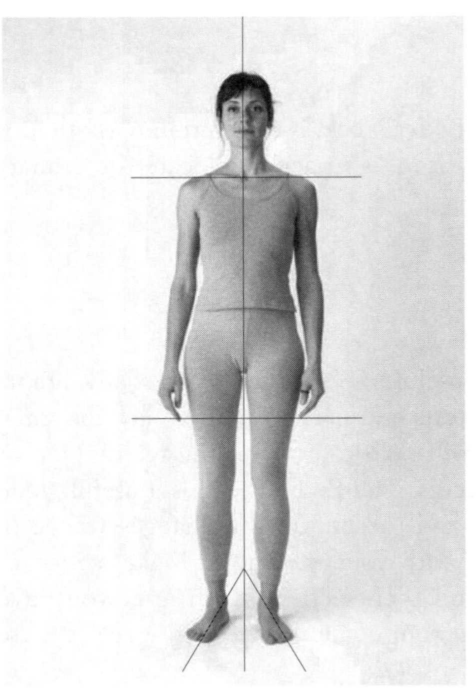

5. How are your knees aligned? Does one seem to stick out in front of the other? What is the alignment of your lower legs?

6. Check the alignment of your feet. Is one rotated in or out in relation to the other? Notice the height of your arches. Is one different from the other?

Neck Ranges of Motion

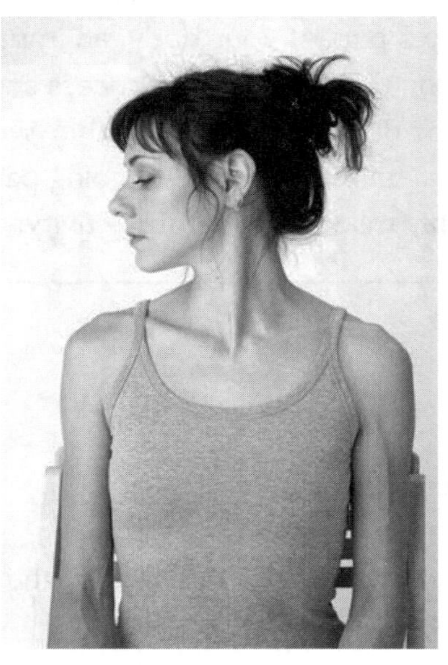

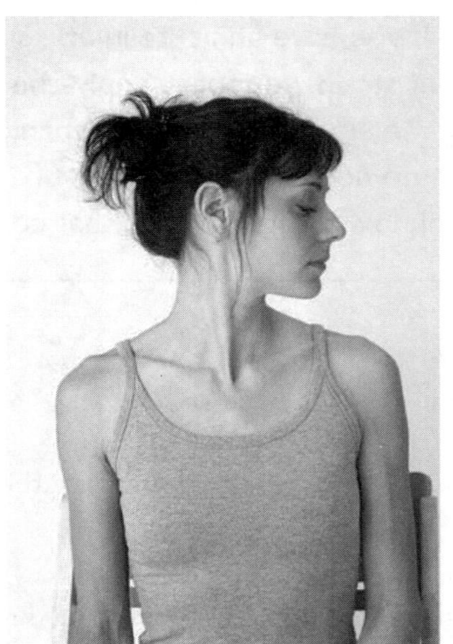

Sit up straight. Turn your head to the right. Notice how far you can trun in relation to your shoulders. Do the same on the left. Notice if there is any discomfort in one direction or the other.

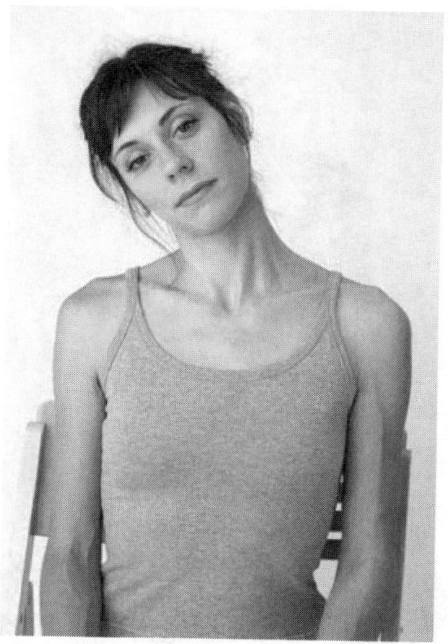

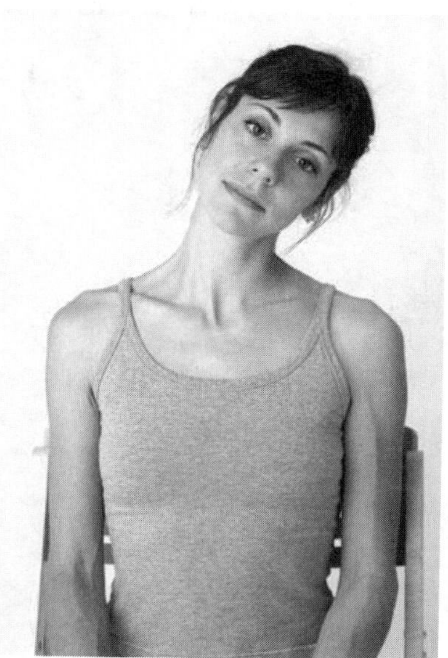

Sit up straight and face a vertical landmark (the corner between two walls or a door frame). Tip your right ear toward your right shoulder. Notice how far you can go in relation to the vertical in each direction. Another method of measurement is to try to fit your hand, or however many fingers will fit, between your shoulder and the side of your head, just below your earlobe. Again, notice if there is any discomfort in either direction.

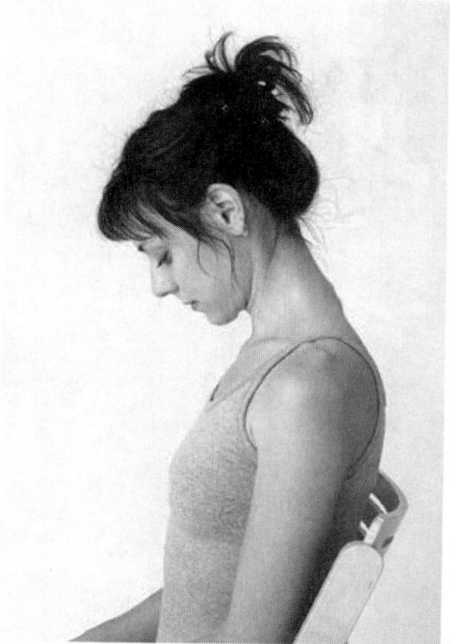

Bend your head forward. Notice how far you can reach your chin toward your chest.

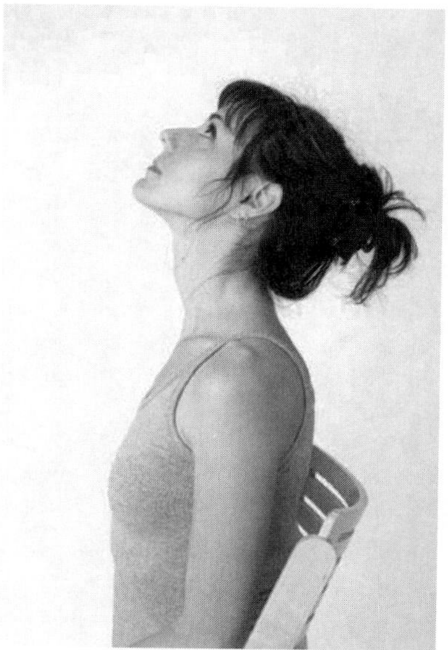

Bend your head gently backward. Notice how far you reach in relation to a spot on the ceiling, staying within your comfort range.

Shoulder, Elbow, Wrist, and Hand Ranges of Motion

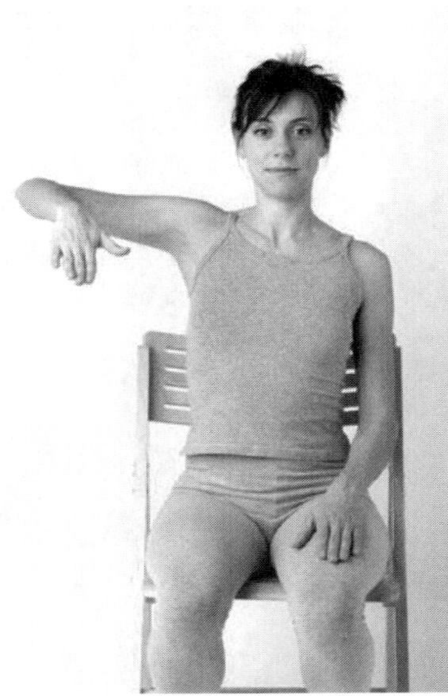

With your arm at your side, bend your elbow 90 degrees so that it is parallel to the floor. Now lift your arm straight out at your side while keeping your arm at this angle. Look to the side or do it in front of a mirror to note how high you can lift your arm. Do this on both sides.

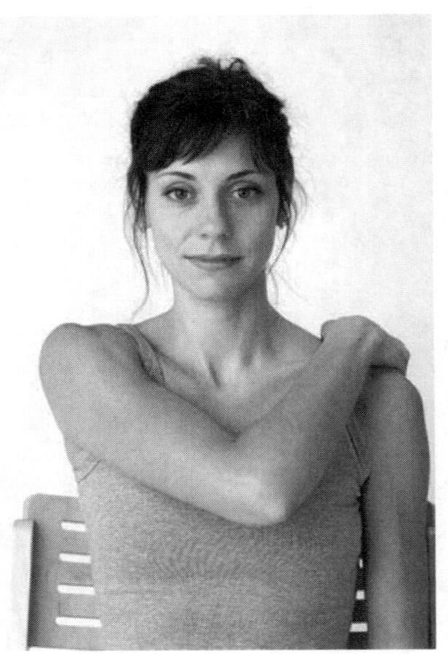

Reach your arm across your chest as far over to the opposite shoulder as you can. Repeat on the opposite side. Notice any differences from one side to the other.

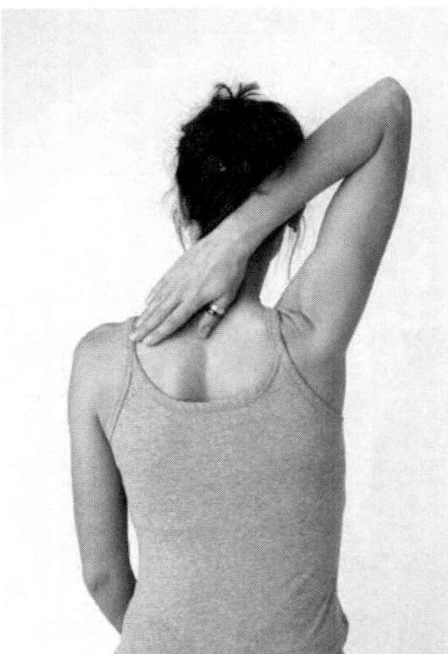

Reach your arm up and behind your head as far over to the opposite shoulder as you can. Repeat on the opposite side. Notice any differences from one side to the other.

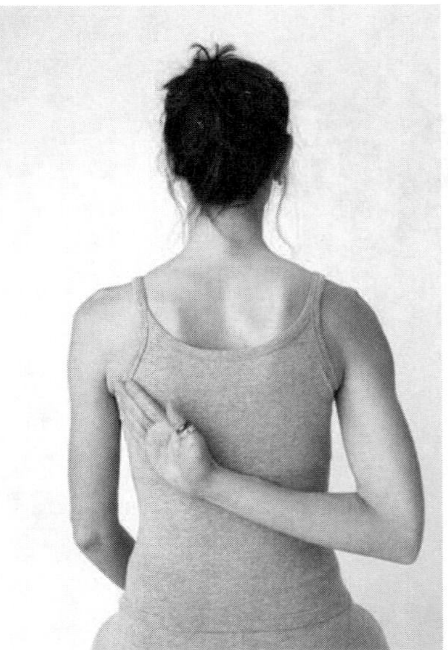

Reach your arm down and behind your back as far up the back as you can. Repeat on the opposite side. Notice any differences from one side to the other.

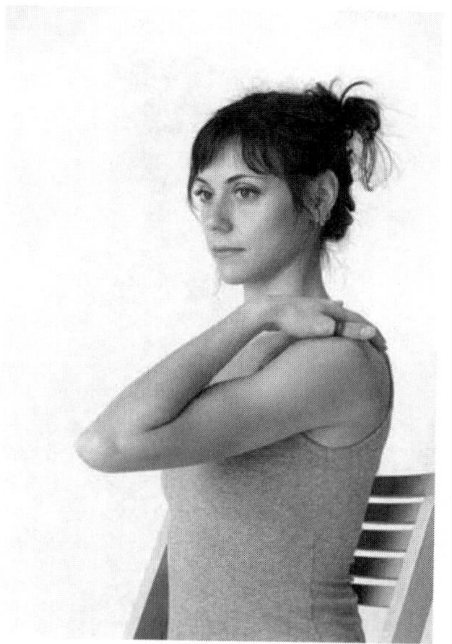

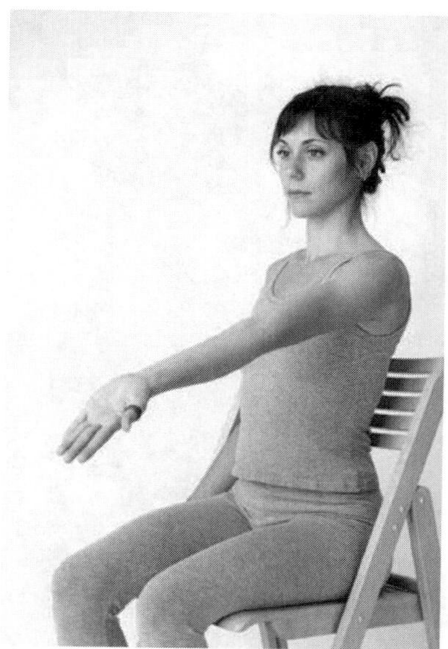

Bend and straighten each elbow fully to check if there are any differences from one side to the other.

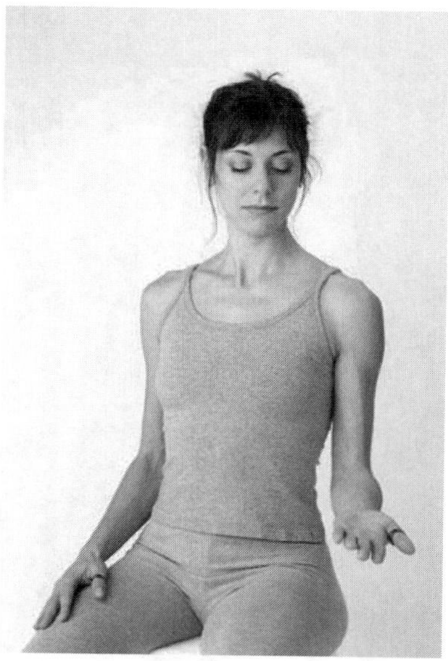

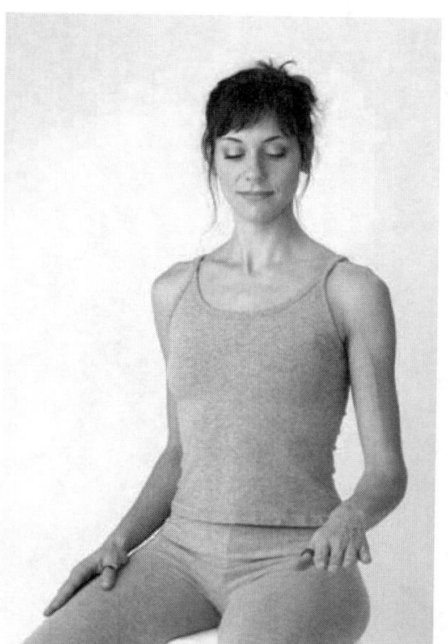

With your arm at your side, the elbow bent at 90 degrees, and the palm of your hand facing to the center, turn your hand so that it is facing palm up and palm down as far as it will go. Repeat on the opposite side, noticing any differences.

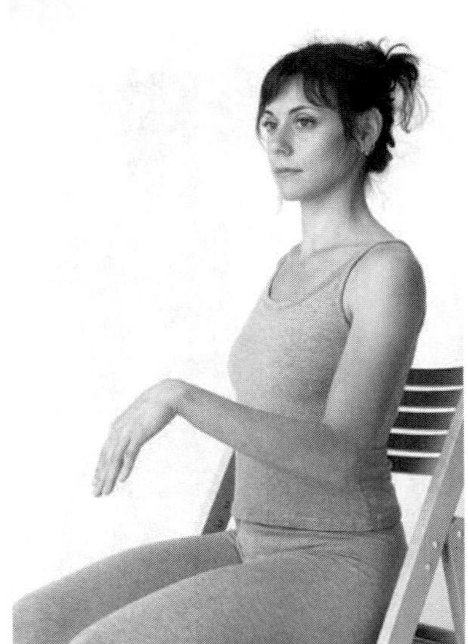

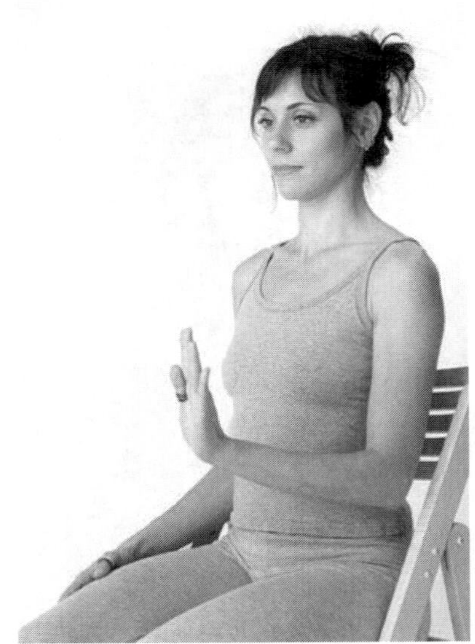

With your arm at your side, the elbow bent at 90 degrees, and the palm of your hand facing toward the floor, bend your wrist as far toward the floor and toward the ceiling as possible. Repeat on the other side and note any limitations or differences from one side to the other.

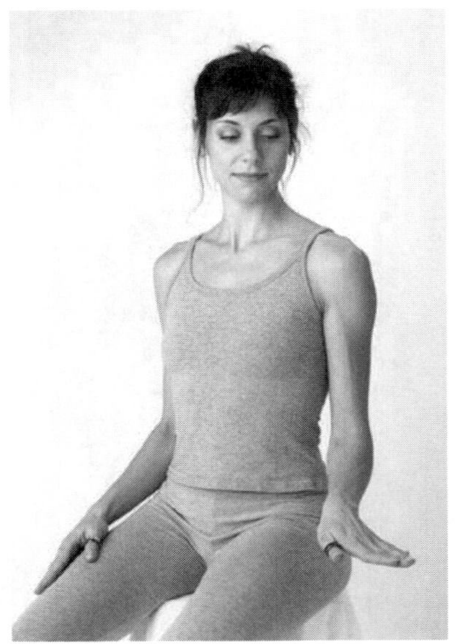

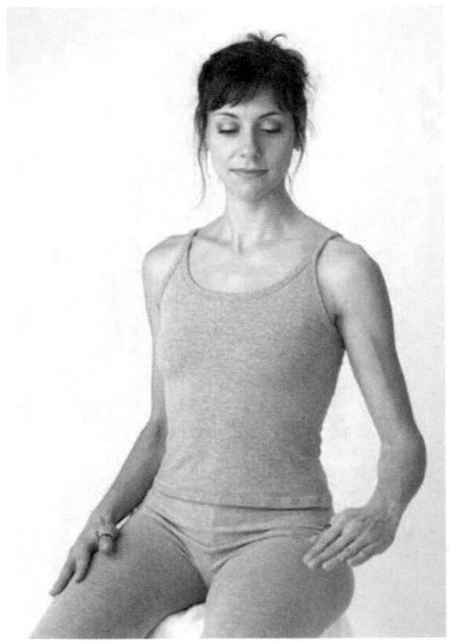

With your arm at your side, the elbow bent at 90 degrees, and the palm of your hand facing toward the floor, bend your wrist as far to the right and as far to the left as possible. Note any limitations or differences from one side to the other.

Low Back Ranges of Motion

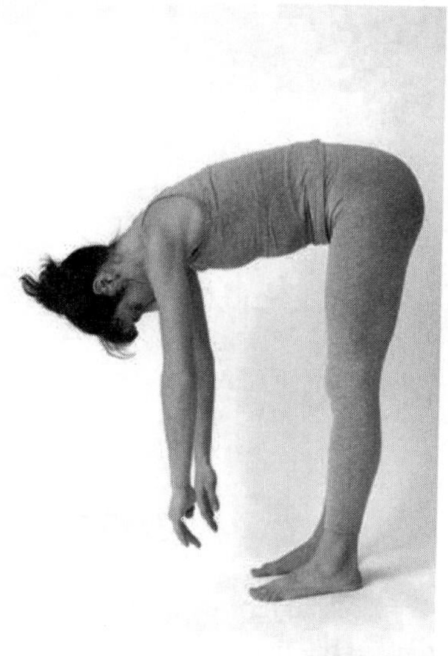

From a standing position, bend over at the waist while keeping your legs straight. Notice how far down your legs you can reach.

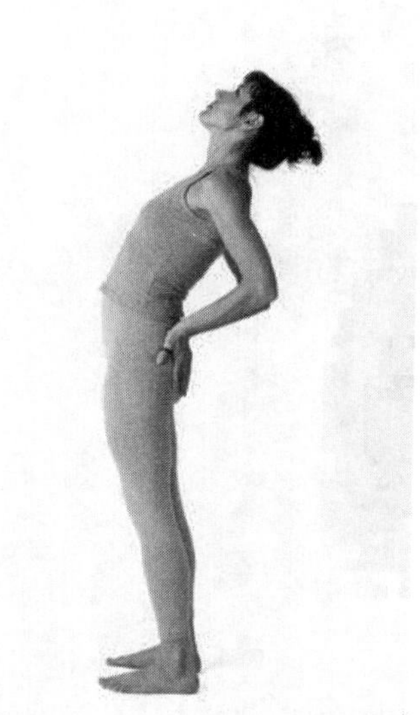

From a standing position, place your hands on the back of your hips and arch backward while looking up at the ceiling. Notice how far you are able to do this comfortably. Use a reference point on the ceiling to measure this range.

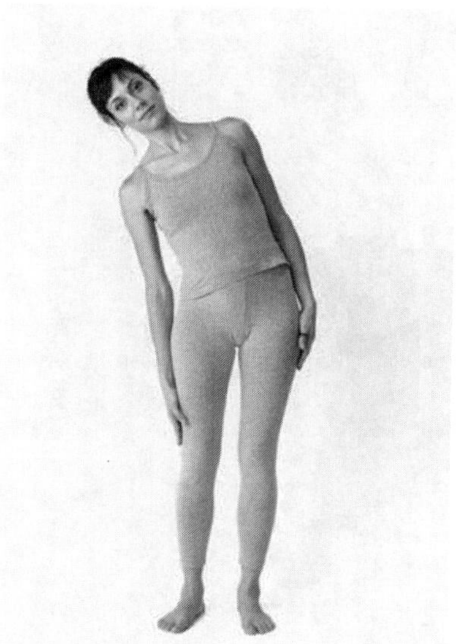

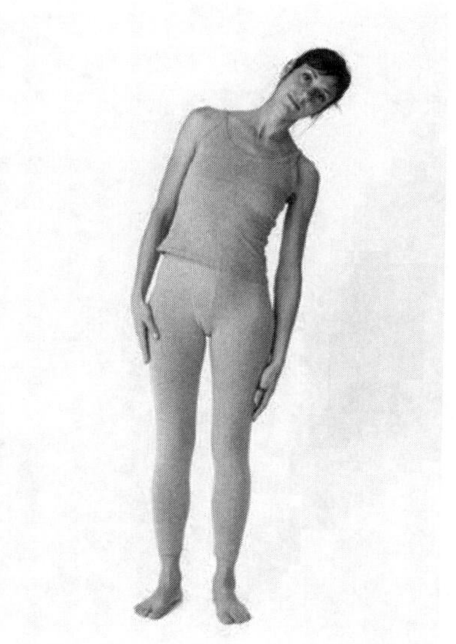

From a standing position, bend sideways to the right. Slide your right arm down the side of your right leg, and notice how far down you can reach. Repeat on the left side.

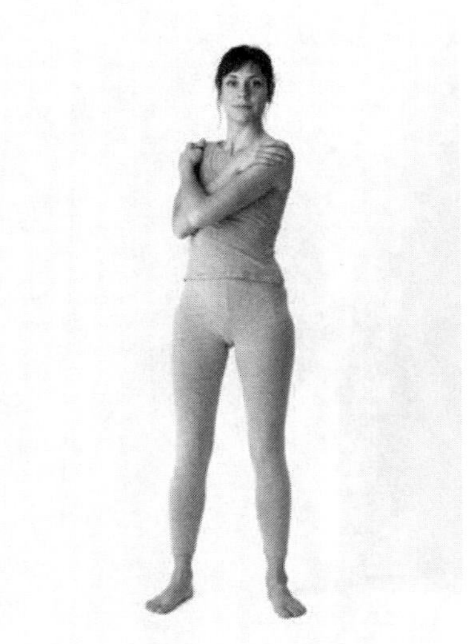

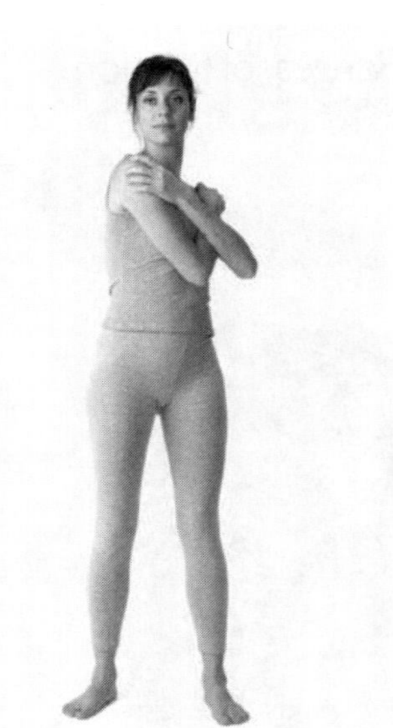

Fold your arms across your chest. Keeping your hips and legs in place, rotate your trunk to the right as far as you can. Keep your head and neck in line with your chest and notice how far you can rotate in relation to a reference point on the wall. Repeat by rotating to the left.

Hip Ranges of Motion

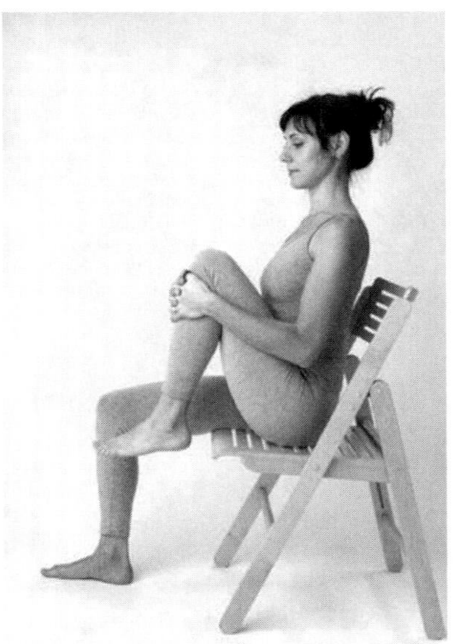

Sit up straight in a chair. Grasp one knee with both your hands and pull it up toward your chest. Notice how far you can move it. Repeat on the opposite side.

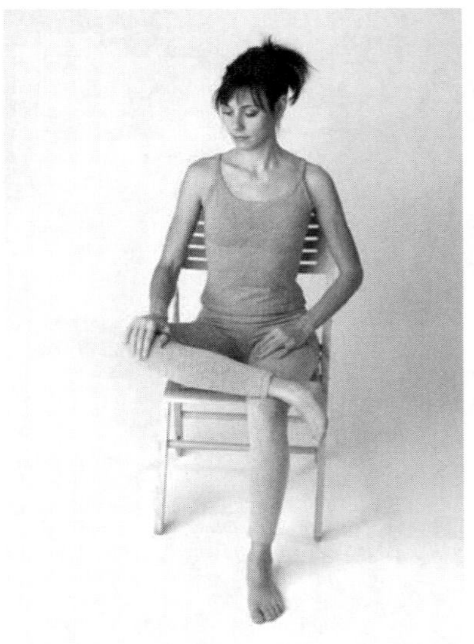

Place the outside of your right foot on top of your left thigh near the knee. Allow your right knee to rotate out to the side. Notice how far it will rotate comfortably. Repeat, using the left leg.

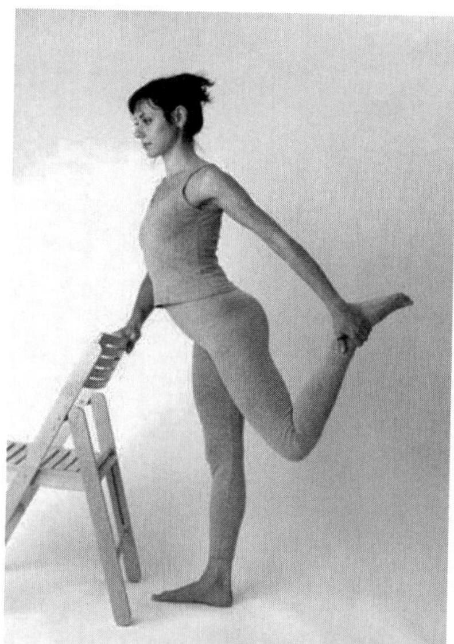

Stand up in front of a full-length mirror and hold on to a support (chair, railing, wall) using your left hand. Bend your right knee, lifting your foot toward your buttocks. With your right hand, grasp the front of your right foot and pull it backward, extending your right hip backward as far as you comfortably can. Look in the mirror and notice how far you can move your hip in this direction. Repeat this for the left hip.

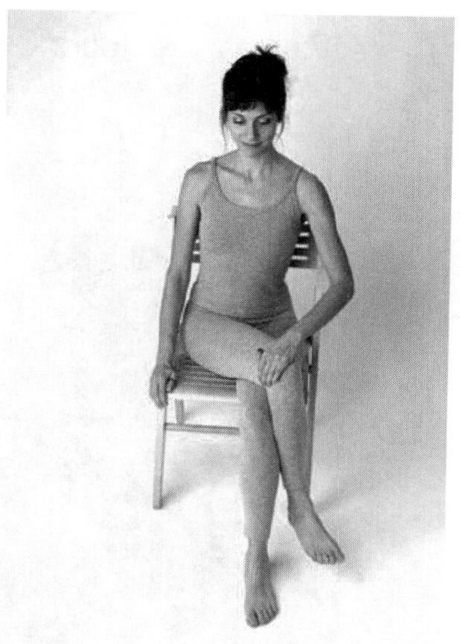

Sit in a chair. Lift one leg and cross it over the other. Grasp the knee of the upper leg and pull it gently to the opposite side. Repeat this for the other leg. Note if one side feels more restricted than the other or if it doesn't move as far.

Knee Ranges of Motion

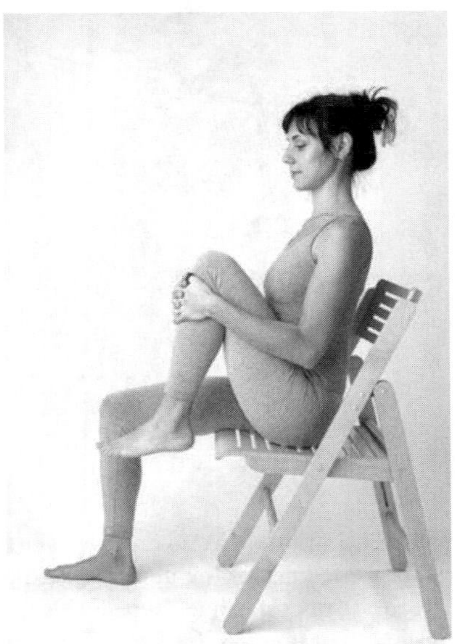

Sit in a chair or lie down. Lift one leg and clasp your hands below the knee. Pull it in, toward the chest. Notice how far you can do this comfortably. Repeat on the opposite side.

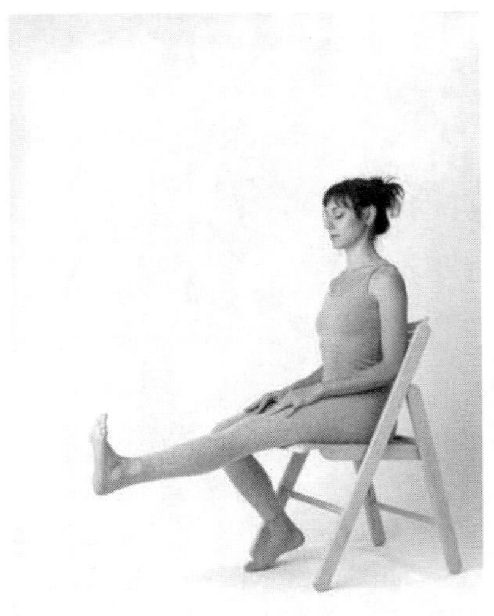

Sit in a chair. Fully straighten one leg out in front of you. Repeat with the other leg. Notice if there is a difference in the amount you can straighten one or the other, or if the position causes any pain in the knee.

Ankle Ranges of Motion

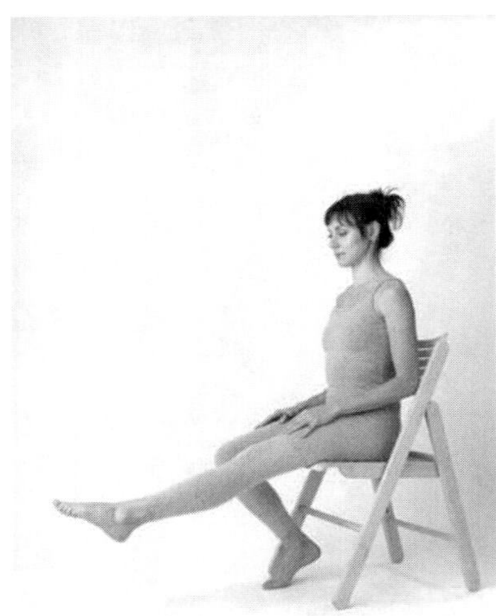

Sit in a chair or lie down. Point one foot at a time away from your head. Notice if there is any difference between the two ankles.

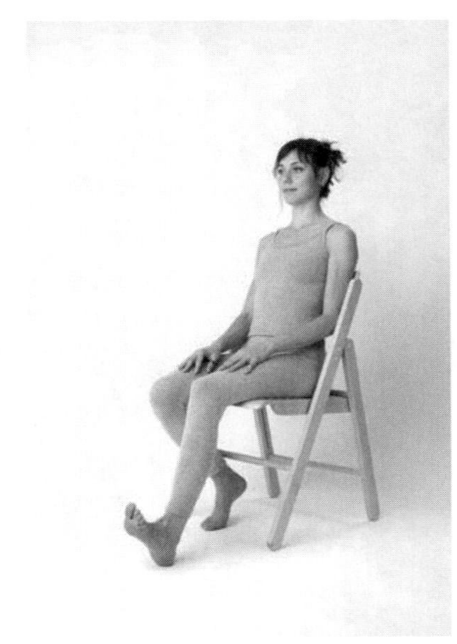

Sit in a chair or lie down. Point one foot at a time toward your head. Notice if there is any difference between the two ankles.

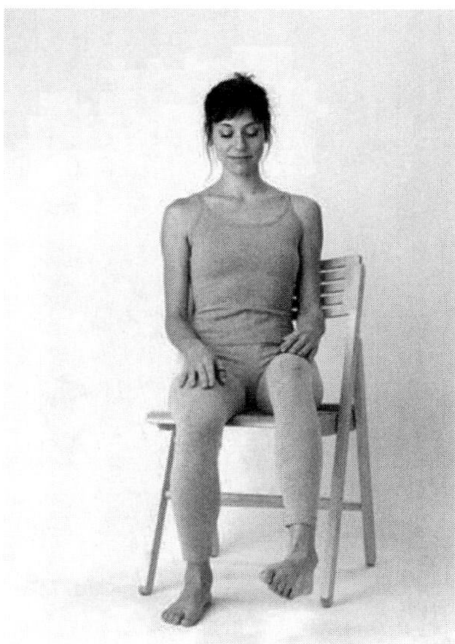

Sit in a chair or lie down. Bend one ankle at a time so the bottom of the foot is facing inward. Notice if there is any difference between the two ankles.

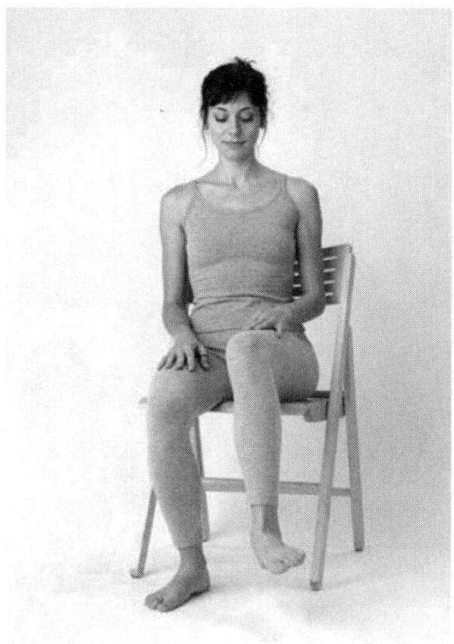

Sit in a chair or lie down. Bend one ankle at a time so the bottom of the foot is facing outward. Notice if there is any difference between the two ankles.

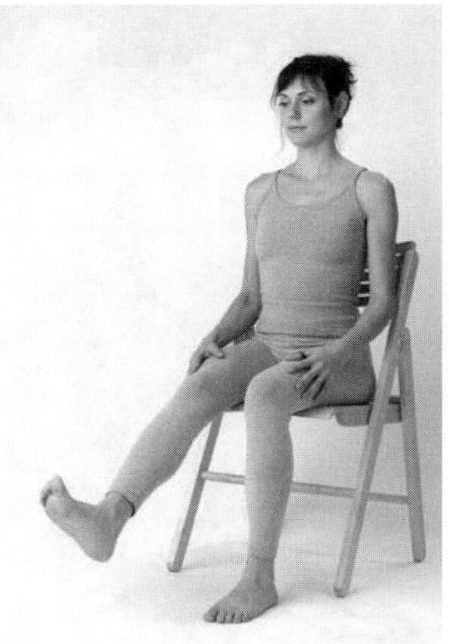

Holding your foot off the ground, rotate your ankle clockwise and counter- clockwise. Repeat with the other foot. Is there any difference in the amount of movement from one ankle to the other?

Foot Ranges of Motion

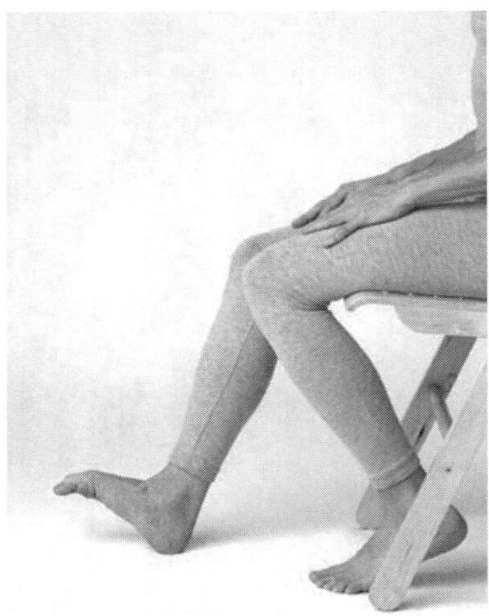

Sitting in a chair, curl the toes of one foot at a time toward the floor. Notice any difference between the two feet.

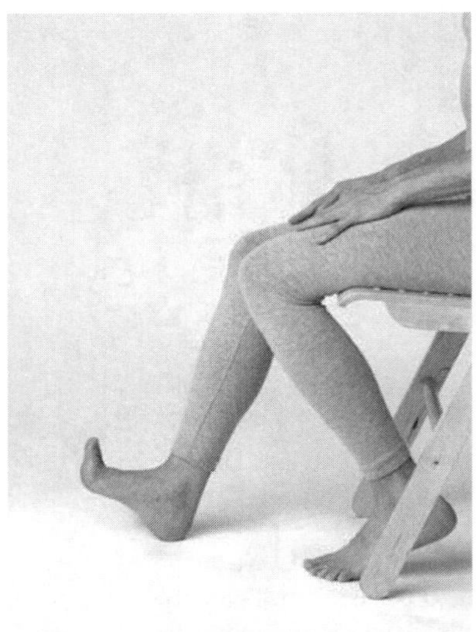

Sitting in a chair, extend the toes of one foot at a time toward your head. Notice any difference between the two feet.

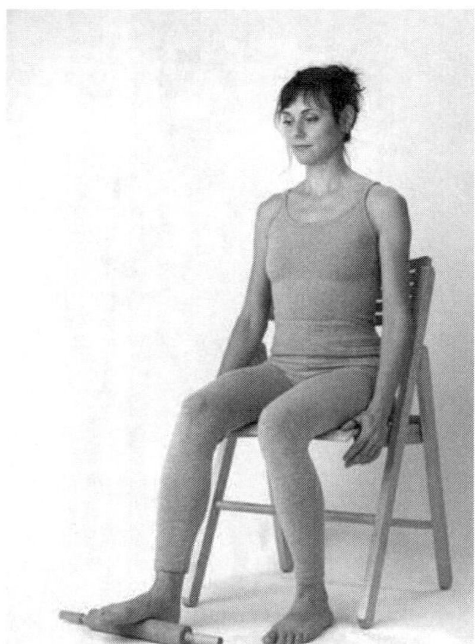

Find a rolling pin or a sturdy bottle about the same diameter as one. Sit in a chair and place one foot on it. Put a comfortable amount of pressure on the rolling pin or bottle and roll your foot forward and backward. Notice how much flexibility there is in your foot and if there is any discomfort doing this. Repeat with the other foot.

Grip Strength

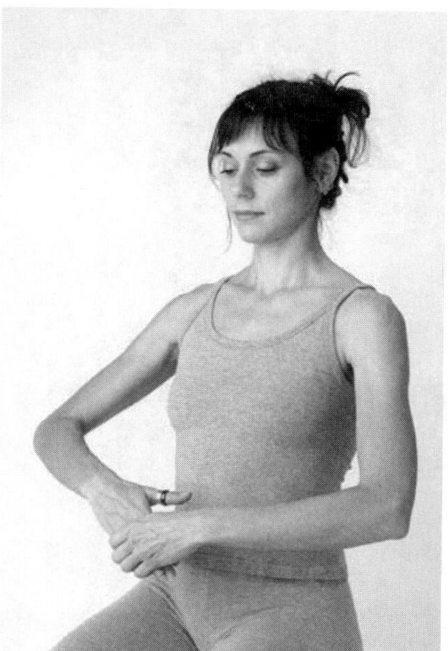

Grasp the fingers of your right hand with your left hand. Squeeze as hard as you can. Repeat, using the left hand on the right wrist. Notice the relative strength of your grip from one hand to the other.

Muscle Tone

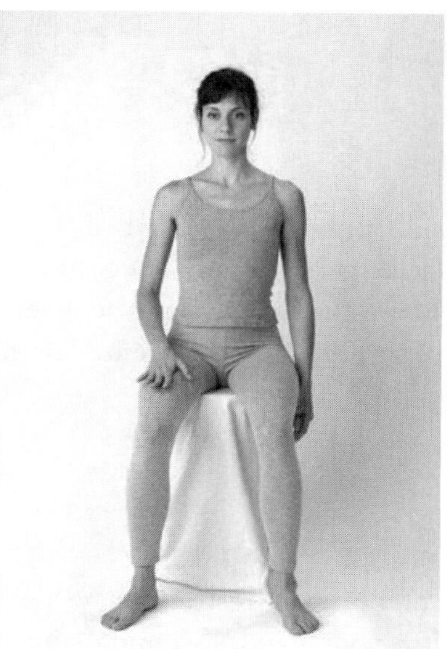

Sit in a chair. Relax your legs. Place your right hand on the muscles of the right thigh. Push gently into the muscle and notice the degree of firmness. Compare this to the opposite side.

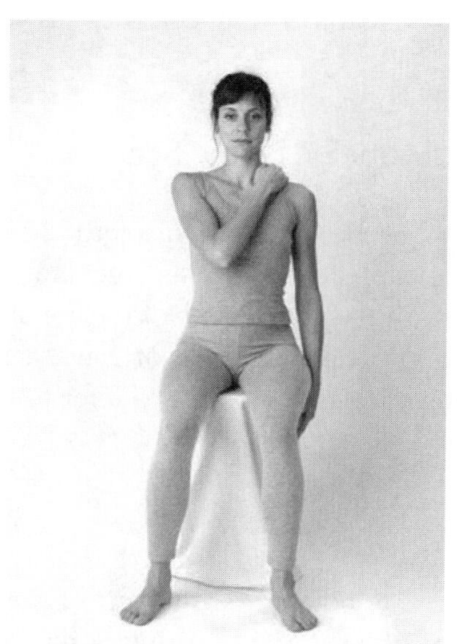

Sitting in a chair, press or squeeze the muscle connecting the neck to the shoulder (trapezius). Compare the tension on one side with the other side.

Facial Symmetry

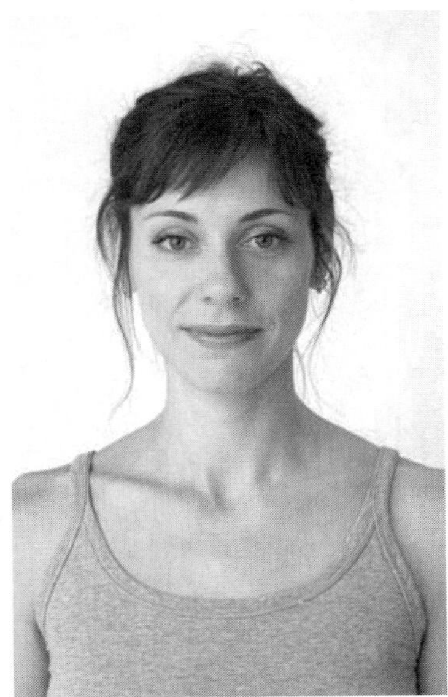

Look at the general shape of your face. Look at the size of each eye, the shape of your cheekbones and forehead, and the position of your lower jaw. Note any asymmetry between the right and left sides. Look at the pupils of both eyes. Notice if there is any difference in size from one side to the other.

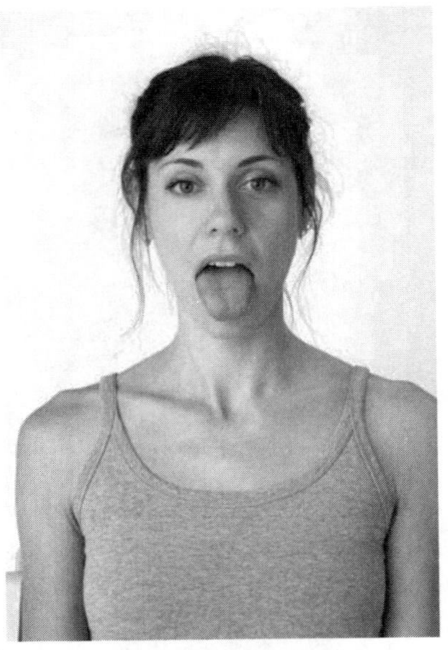

Stick out your tongue. Does it angle to one side or the other?

Surgery and other Scars

These areas are often associated with abnormal tension in the body. Make a note of their location so you remember to check them as you scan your body.

Step 2: Body Scan

The Body Scan is a method to locate areas of primary restriction throughout your body. A total body scan can be used as a general self-checkup, which you may want to perform only once, just to see where the major sources of tension are located. However, many people use the Body Scan whenever they develop a new problem or have a problem that has not responded to previous treatment. For many minor injuries, you can also refer to the areas listed in chapter 6.

The Indicator

The indicator is any part of the body used to verify the location of a primary restriction. When your hand is placed over a primary restriction, the normal electrical field in your hand, assuming your hand has not been seriously injured (if it is, see the section on treatment of the hand in chapter 5), will tend to shift the molecules in the area of the primary restriction toward their normal, relaxed state. Since the matrix forms a continuous fabric throughout the body, a reduction in tension in the primary restriction will reduce tension everywhere else. Therefore, by feeling for the softening (see: The Resistance Barrier, below) of the indicator, you can precisely locate the primary restrictions anywhere else in the body. The indicator will also be used in the Treatment section to verify the completion of the treatment.

Any part of the body may be used as an indicator. Two different indicators are described in this book: the thigh muscle and the fingers. We have found these two parts of the body to be the easiest to use for the Body Scan, but you may find that another part of your body is more accessible in different situations. The only stipulation is that, no matter which area you use as the indicator, you compare the change in tension there with your other hand over the potential primary restriction (target area) and then with your other hand away from the target area. A primary restriction is verified if there is a greater degree of softening of the indicator with your hand over the target compared with your hand away from the target. This is the key to locating the source of the problem and where to treat it.

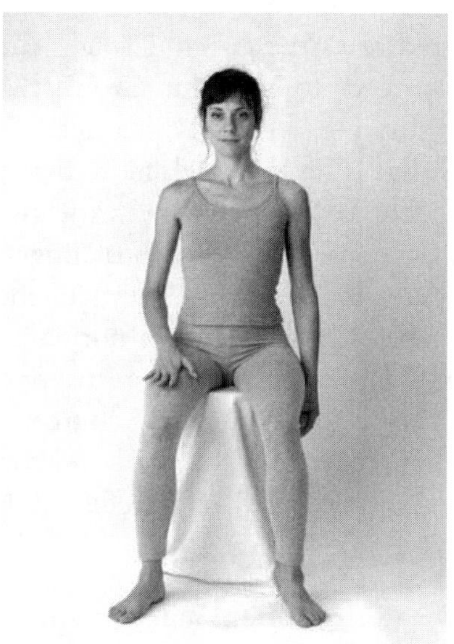

Thigh muscle pressure test

Thigh Muscle Pressure Test

1. While seated, place the palm of one hand on top of the center of your thigh on the same side. For example, right hand on right thigh or left hand on left thigh.

2. Press down gently on the center of your thigh muscles with your hand pushing toward the floor.

Finger Bend Test

1. Gently push one finger or your thumb in toward the palm of your hand using another finger or the thumb in the same hand.

2. Notice the degree to which you can push your fingers or thumb.

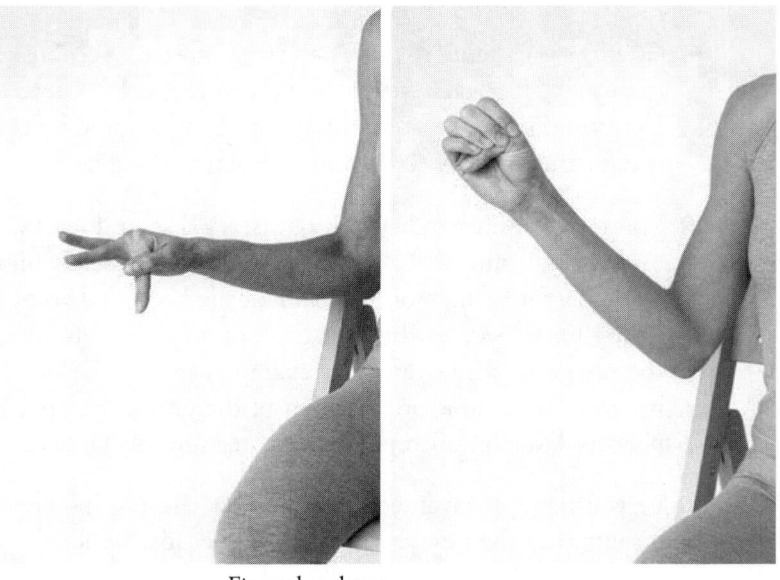

Finger bend test

Using the Indicator

1. With either of the tests outlined above, get a sense of how much you have to push or squeeze until you meet resistance. Only use mild pressure until you feel a *slight* resistance in the muscle or in the joints of the finger or thumb. You will notice a natural stopping point where the pressure of your hand or fingers and the resistance you are pushing against are about equal. This is referred to as the *resistance barrier* (see below).

2. Rest your hand on your thigh without pressing down or place your fingers and thumb gently against each other without pushing.

3. Place your other hand over or touch each body part, one by one, as listed on pages [65, 66]. The hand used to contact the various parts of the body is referred to as the *targeting hand*. The targeting hand does not actually have to touch the area—it only needs to be within two inches of the part you are testing. You can test these areas through clothing, so there's no need to disrobe. After you contact each area, press down with the hand that is on the thigh more firmly into the muscle or push gently on your thumb or finger. Notice if there is any change in the *give* or softness in the thigh muscle or in the ease with which you can push your thumb or finger. What you are looking for is an increase in the give in the indicator muscle or the joints of the hand. When you place your targeting hand over a primary restriction, it will tend to normalize the electrical field in that part. When this happens, the molecules within the primary restriction will shift back toward their normal, more flexible state, which in turn will reduce this source of restriction. Since the matrix connects all parts together, as it relaxes, the whole body relaxes slightly. The indicator (in this case the thigh muscles or joints of the hand) will reflect this change by becoming more relaxed.

4. If placing your hand over any of the target areas causes the indicator to soften, make a note of it.

5. If softening occurs in more than one area, go back and forth to see which of the targets causes the *greatest* amount of softening in the indicator.

6. Confirm with tenderness. The area of greatest response to the indicator is usually very tender to the touch. If it isn't, you may wish to recheck to determine which area is the primary problem. Determining the most significant area takes some practice, so don't be dismayed if you don't get it right the first few times. One adage to remember: "If it isn't sore, explore some more!"

7. You may switch hands when necessary. If you do switch hands, be sure to determine the barrier in the thigh muscle or the hand once again before moving to the next target area. If you are checking for an area on the back of the body and you cannot reach it easily, simply flip your targeting hand over so that the back of your hand is contacting the front of the body across from the area you are testing. For example, to test the back of the chest, turn the hand over so the back of the hand is on the front of the chest. We speculate that this works due to the electrical polarity (North/South pole) characteristics of the body.

Once you have determined which area is causing the greatest change in the indicator, refer to the treatment section in the next chapter for further instructions.

Here's a Hint: If you think you can't possibly do this or feel these subtle changes, let me assure you that *you can!* We have successfully taught this technique to hundreds of people from age of eight to ninety-eight. Relax and let your body tell you where the trouble is and what you can do to help. Trust yourself, and trust your body.

The Resistance Barrier

The resistance barrier is the state of tension present within the body as measured by the degree of "give" in any one particular area. It is the sum total of all of the primary restrictions in the body, due to the interconnected nature of the matrix. The resistance barrier is detected by manual pressure or stress on a part of the body. This is applied gradually until a slight opposing resistance is felt. In the case of pressure, this will feel like the body is gently pushing back at your hand. In the case of stress on a joint, for example, the feeling will be one of tension in the opposite direction to the force applied. A change in the resistance barrier will occur when the targeting hand (see above) is over a primary restriction, or when a treatment is completed (see under Treatment in the next chapter). The resistance barrier may be monitored with the indicator *or* in the area being treated, since they are both connected through the matrix.

TARGET AREAS

Use these photos to guide you in checking your target areas.

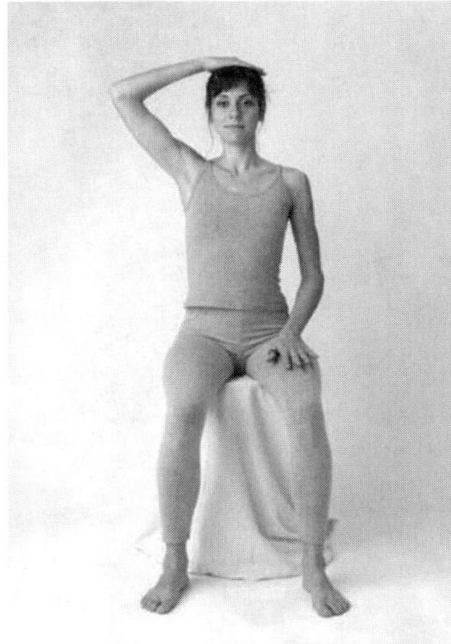

Top of head

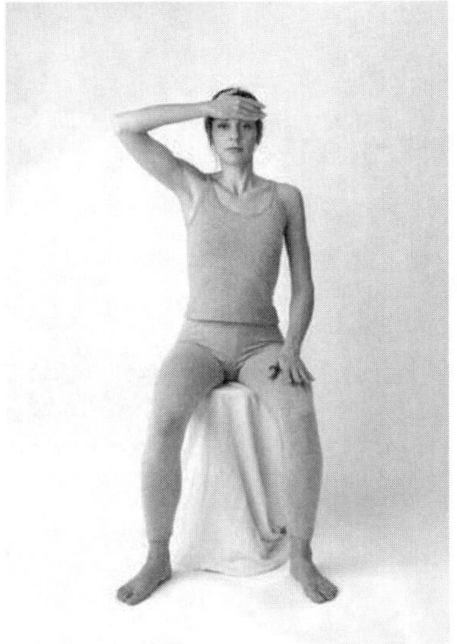

Forehead

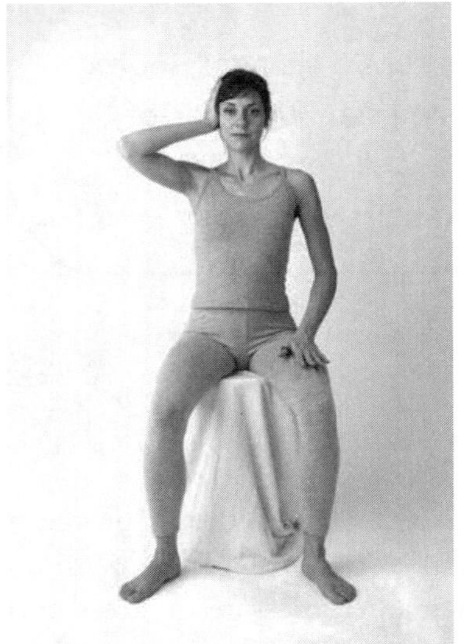

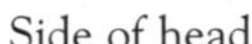

Side of head

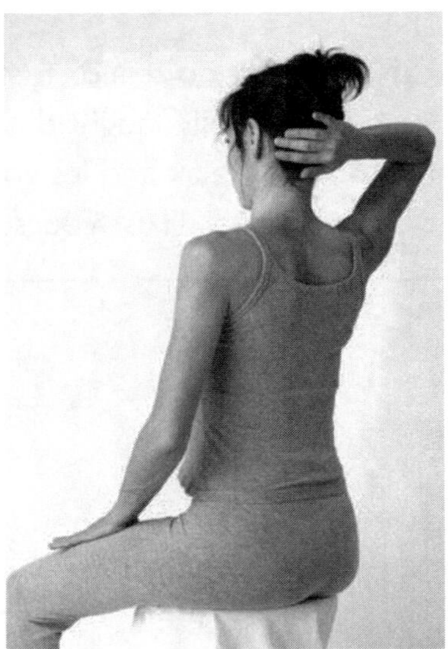

Back of head

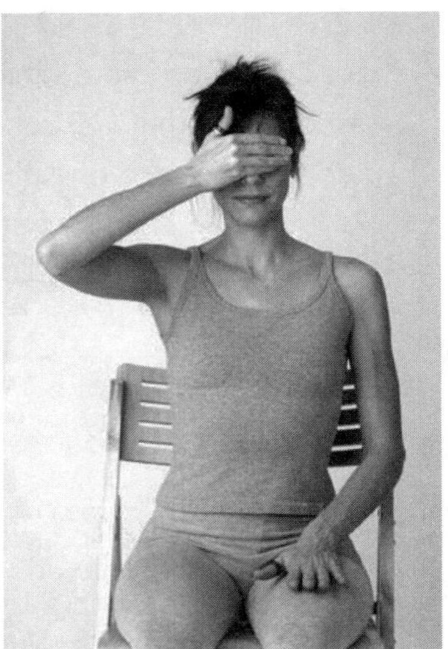

Upper face

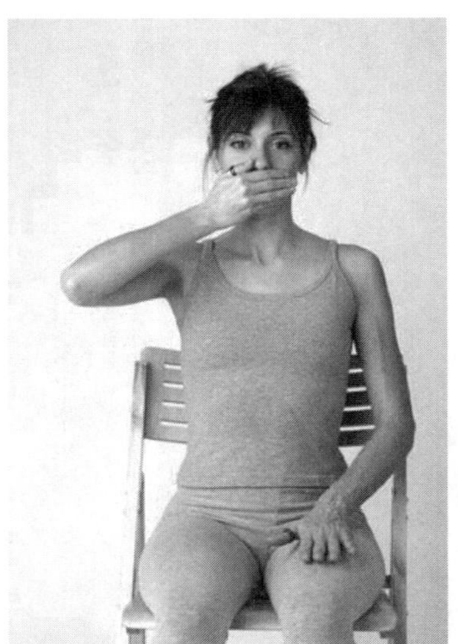

Lower face

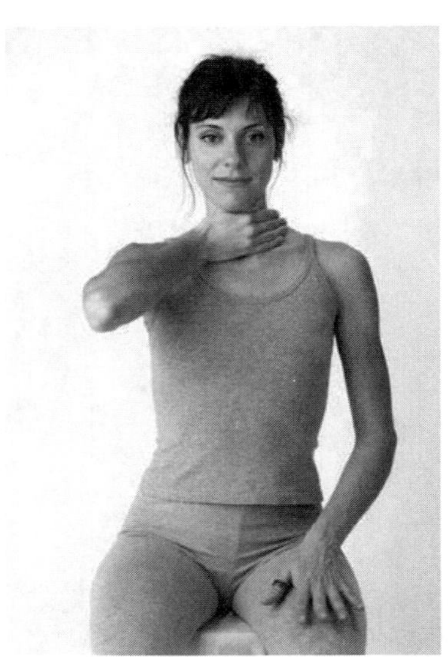

Throat (front of neck)

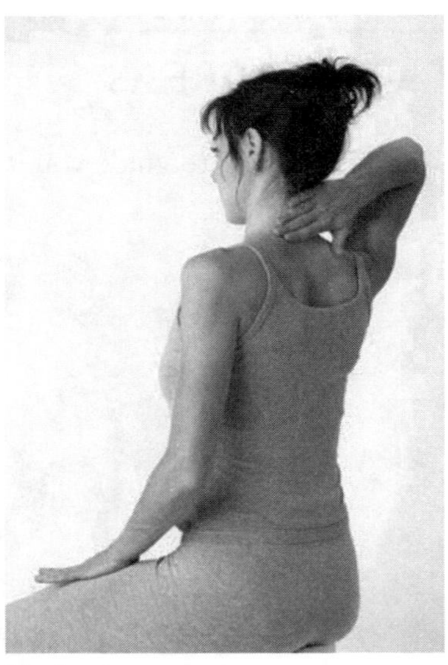

Neck

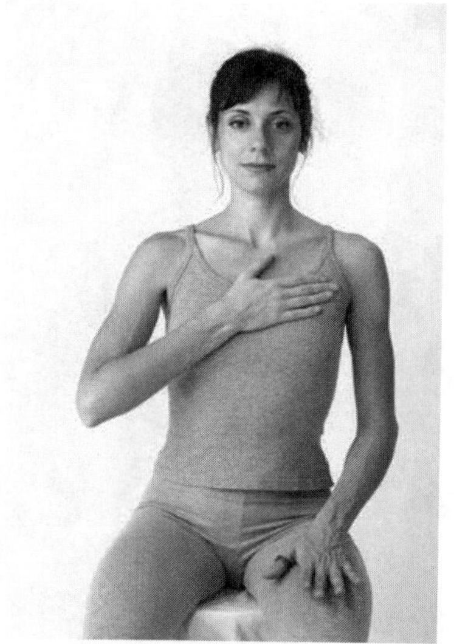
Upper chest (front)

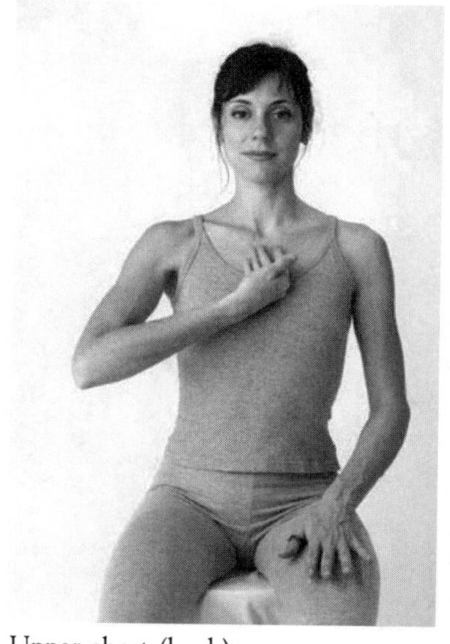
Upper chest (back)

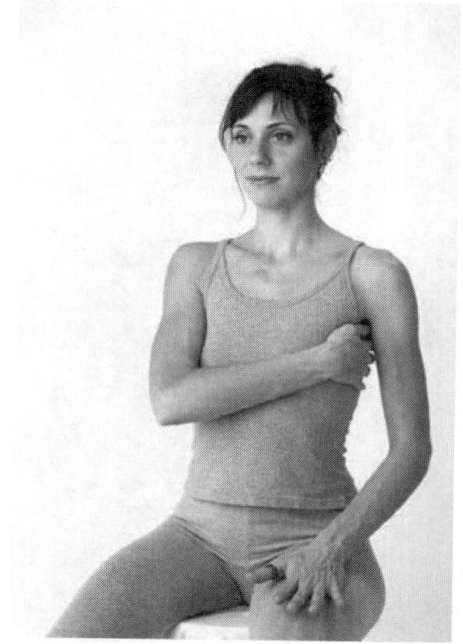
Upper chest (side)

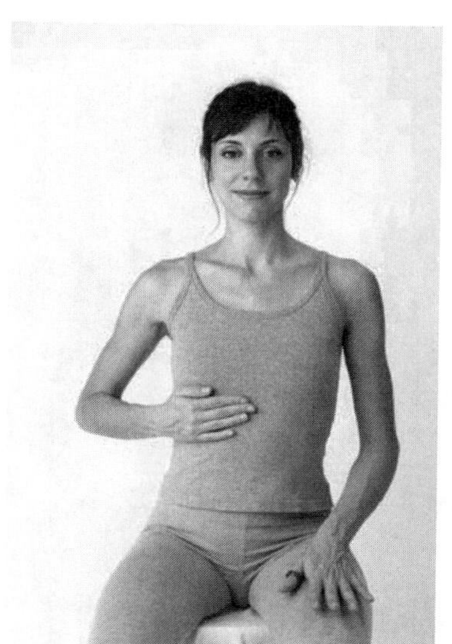
Lower chest (front)

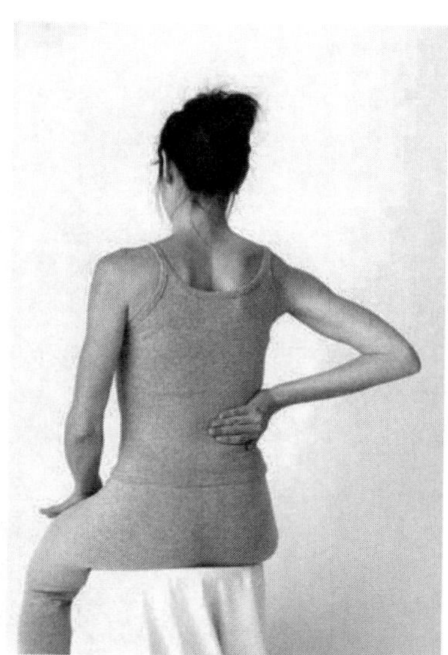
Lower chest (back)

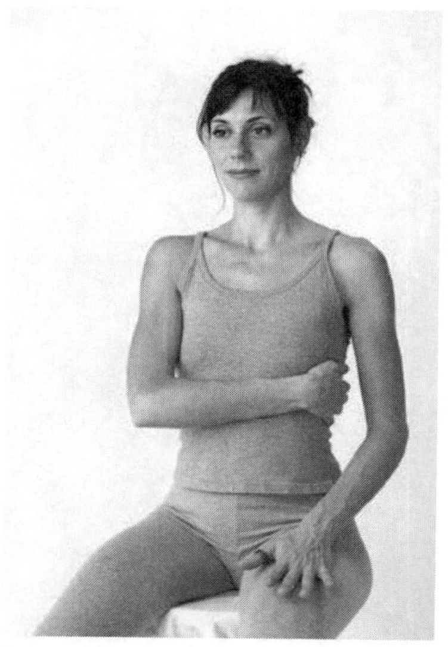
Lower chest (side)

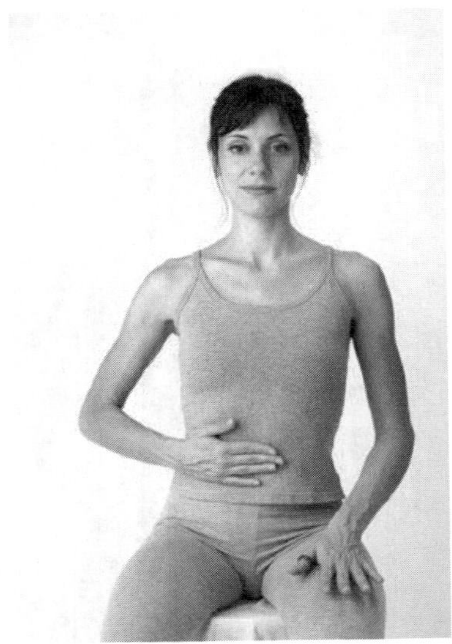

Upper abdomen
front side (right and left)

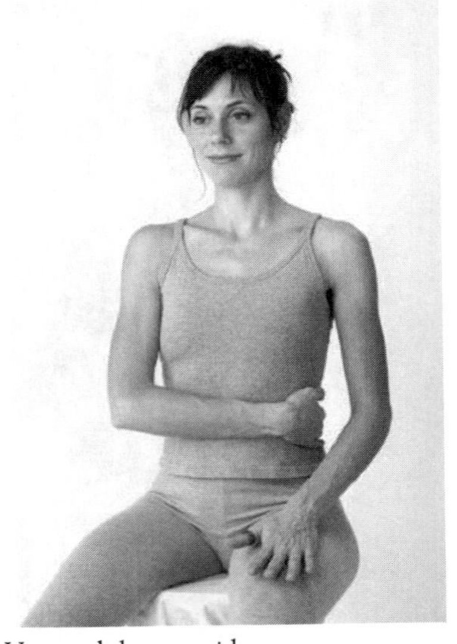

Upper abdomen, side
(right and left)

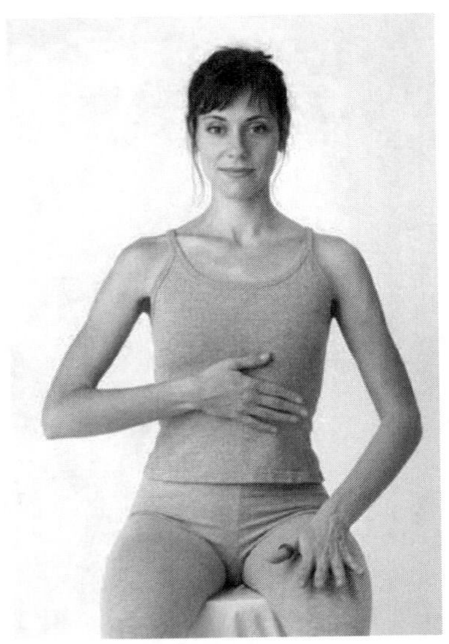

Upper abdomen (center, front)

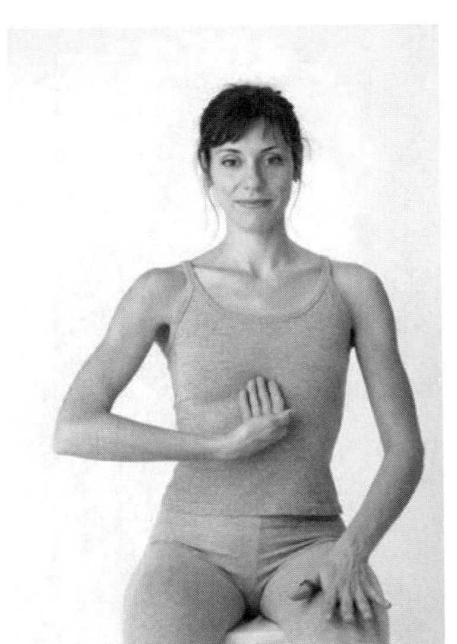

Upper abdomen (center, back)

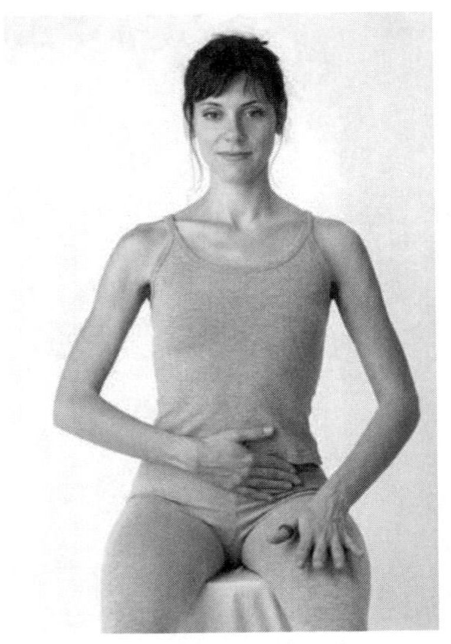

Lower abdomen (center front)

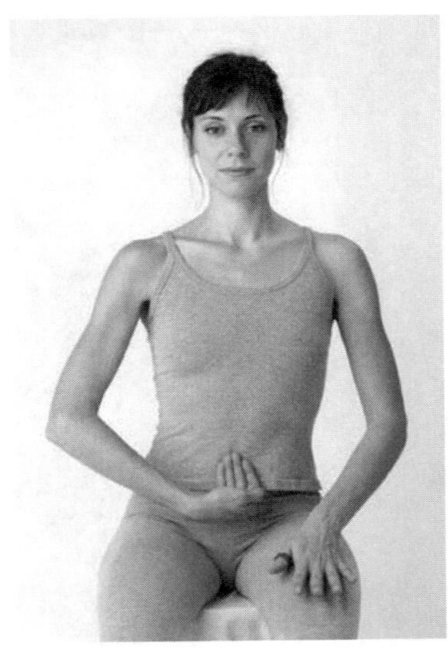

Lower abdomen (back)

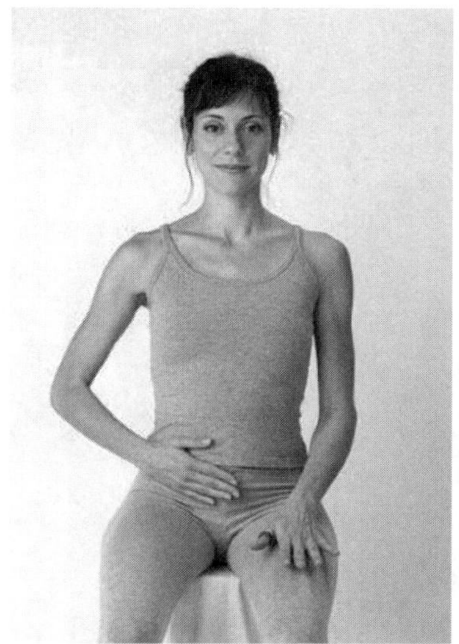

Lower abdomen,
front side (right and left)

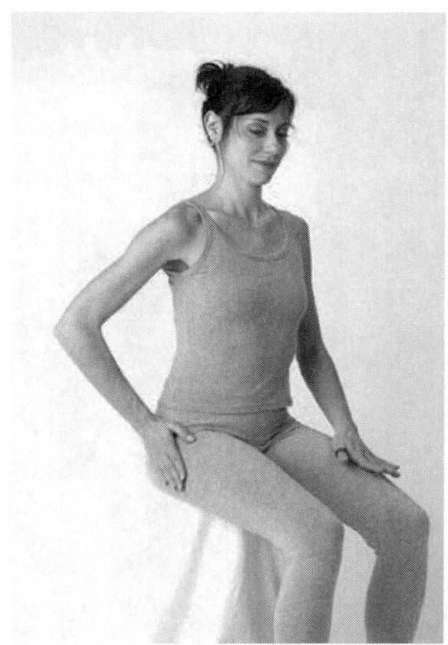

Pelvis side (right and left)

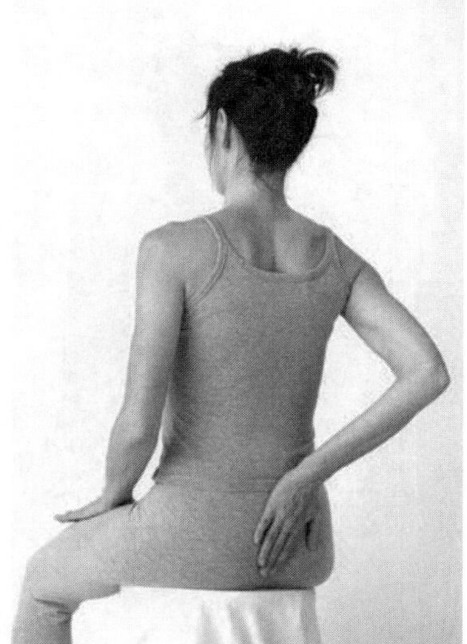

Pelvis (back)

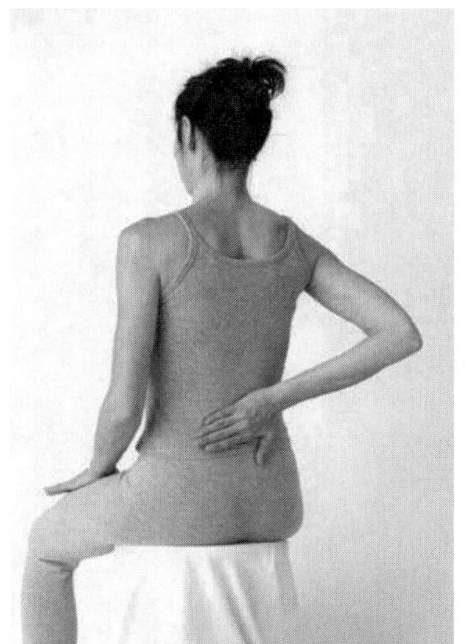

Low back

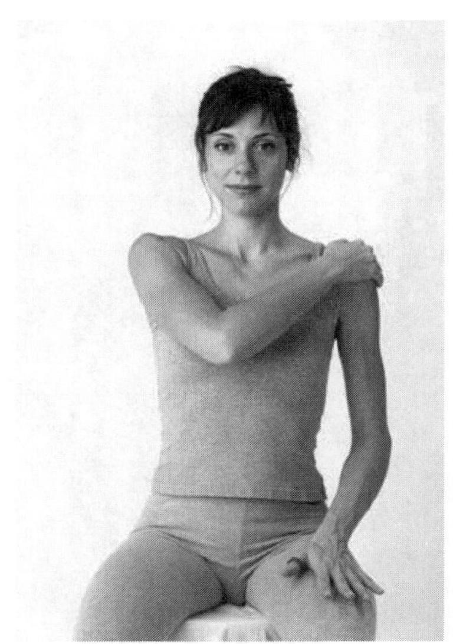

Shoulder

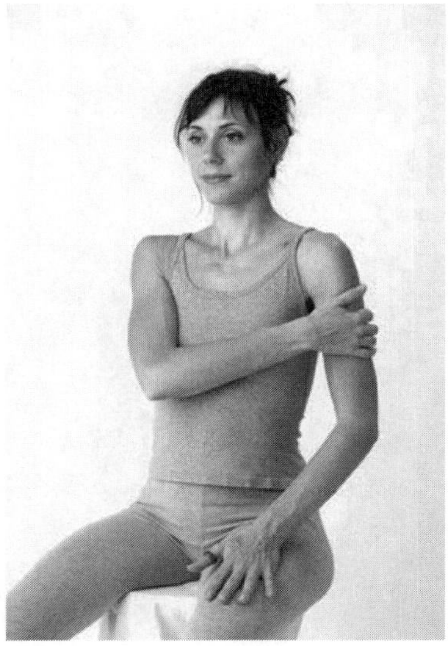

Upper arm

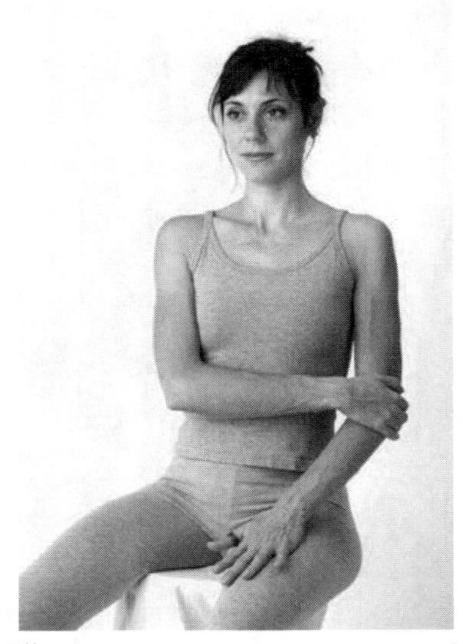

Elbow

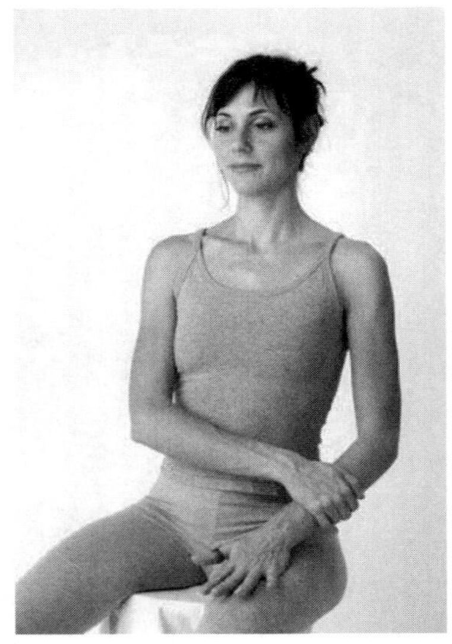
Forearm

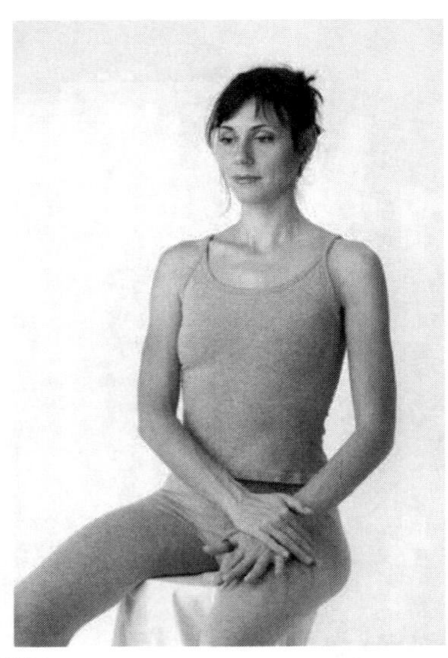
Wrist

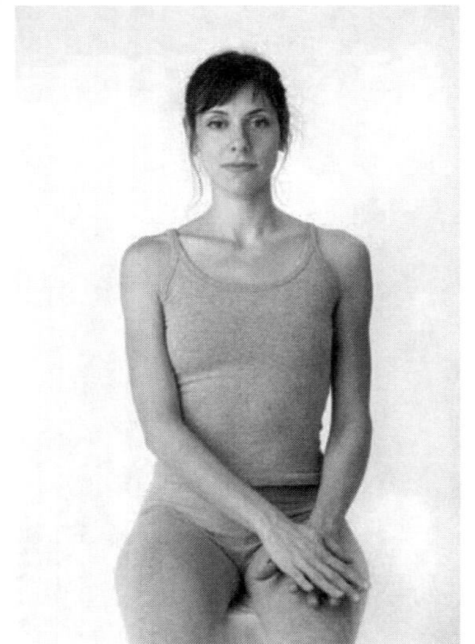
Hand

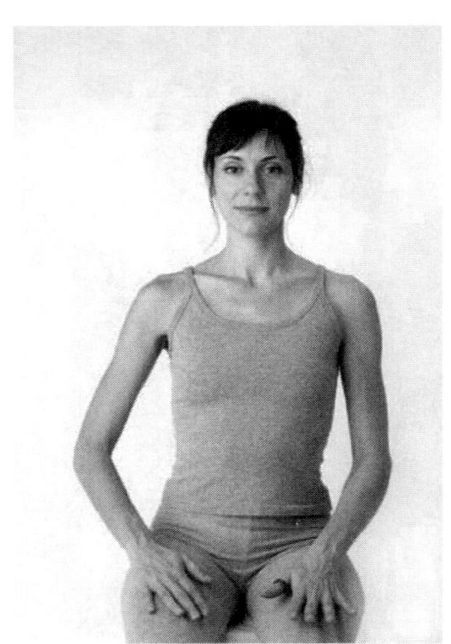
Thigh

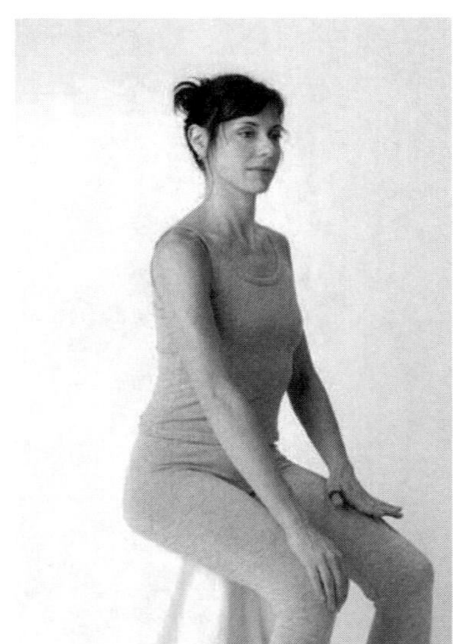
Knee

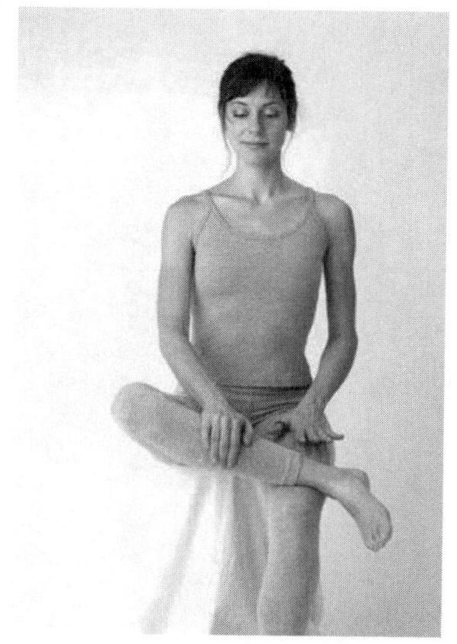
Leg

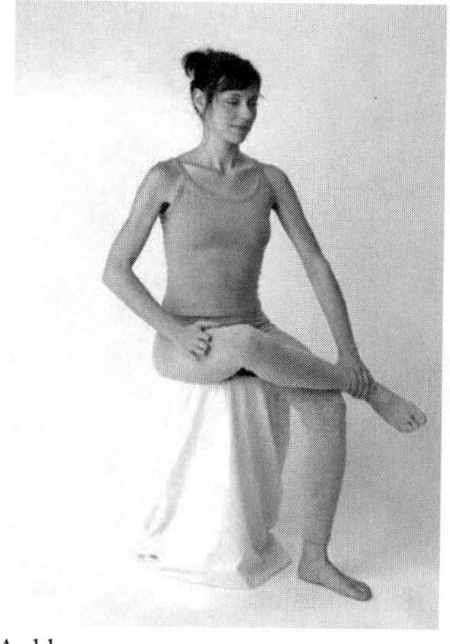
Ankle

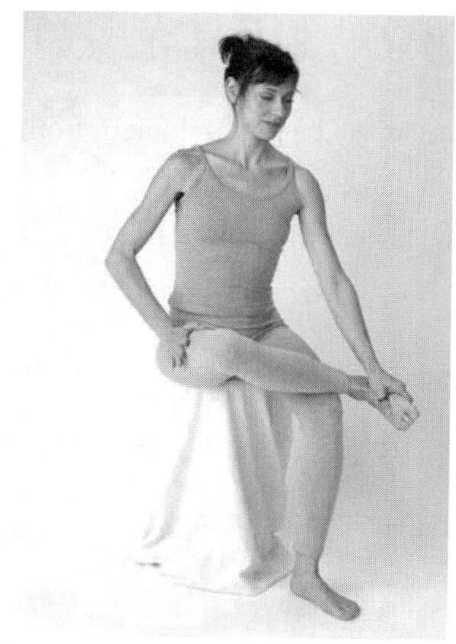
Foot

Summary of Scanned Body Parts

- Top of head
- Forehead
- Side of head
- Back of head
- Upper face
- Lower face
- Throat
- Neck
- Upper chest, front
- Upper chest, back
- Upper chest, side
- Lower chest, front
- Lower chest, back

- Lower chest, side
- Upper abdomen, front side (right and left)
- Upper abdomen, side (right and left)
- Upper abdomen, center, front
- Upper abdomen, center, back
- Lower abdomen, center, front
- Lower abdomen, center, back
- Lower abdomen, front side (right and left)
- Pelvis, side (right and left)
- Pelvis, back
- Low back

Hint: To check the upper limb, use the indicator on the same side as the limb that is being tested.

- Shoulder (right and left)
- Upper arm (right and left)
- Elbow (right and left)
- Forearm (right and left)
- Wrist (right and left)
- Hand (right and left)
- Thigh (right and left)
- Knee (right and left)

Hint: To check the leg, ankle, and foot, rest the lower shin of the side you are testing on the opposite thigh.

- Leg (right and left)
- Ankle (right and left)
- Foot (right and left)
- Scars

Determining Priorities

Once you have determined where the primary restrictions are located, go back and compare the response of the indicator to each primary restriction. See which one causes the greatest softening of the indicator. Remember, your pain could be due to a primary restriction in a totally different part of the body than where you feel pain. Keep an open mind to determine which primary restriction is the most significant.

As you go back and forth between different primaries, you may notice that one or more of them seems to stop affecting the indicator. This is because each time you put your hand over a primary restriction, you are providing a small amount of treatment (see chapter 5). The primary restriction that causes the greatest degree of softening of the indicator is the area that should be treated first. Once this is completed, then go on to the next most significant primary restriction, and so on.

By following the guidelines in chapter 5, you will be able to systematically resolve many of the underlying sources of structural imbalance and the pain they may be causing.

CHAPTER 5

Matrix Repatterning Self-Treatment

This chapter will provide you with simple self-treatment methods to help restore the normal, balanced state of the tensegrity matrix. The result of this will be to reduce strain throughout your body and restore optimal mechanical function in joints and muscles. This self-treatment program is, by definition, a first-aid program that can resolve many minor bumps and strains that you may encounter in day-to-day work, sports, and play activities. Conditions that persist or that don't respond within a reasonable amount of time may require the intervention of a health professional (see appendix 3).

CONDITIONS ASSOCIATED WITH STRUCTURAL IMBALANCE

Joints, muscles, and ligaments are designed to give way when they are strained. They may be directly injured or become painful as a compensation for a restriction in a deeper, denser structure. Because of

When you encounter an injury, you can use the language of the body to easily determine the source of the imbalance. You can then apply the gentle forms of treatment described in this book to encourage the internal structure of your cells back to their balanced state, thus restoring their ideal state of resilience and function.

their density, internal organs and bones absorb more of the energy of impact injuries. Injuries can cause the fibrous tissue around the organs and the fibrous framework within the bones to become restricted and deformed. Strain patterns result in a complex, interconnecting network of abnormal tension leading to many painful and imbalanced conditions of the body, which may contribute to some of the following:

- Arthritis
- Fibromyalgia
- Back and neck pain
- Imbalanced posture and abnormal curvature of the spine
- Hip pain
- Knee pain
- Foot problems or fallen arches
- Shoulder, arm, or hand pain
- Tennis elbow
- Carpal tunnel syndrome
- Symptoms of numbness, tingling, or weakness
- Restricted movement
- Unstable joints
- Heart and respiratory problems
- Digestive complaints
- Reproductive system disorders
- Menstrual pain
- Headaches and migraines
- Temporomandibular joint syndrome (TMJ)
- Tooth pain
- Dizziness and ear noise
- Sleep problems

WHAT YOU'RE GOING TO LEARN

Matrix Repatterning Self-Treatment consists of the following components:

- Electrical Treatment to help restore the normal electrical field within the primary restriction
- Mechanical Treatment to help reverse the mechanical effects of certain injuries
- Simple measures to help family members with minor injuries
- Suggestions for applying the treatment principles into your lifestyle

The goal of Matrix Repatterning is always to move the body towards a more balanced state of normal tone by restoring the natural, relaxed state of the molecular structure. It is therefore virtually impossible, once the correction is completed, to overtreat since it is now in a restored, stable configuration. The only concern is that the wrong area may be treated, in which case little or no positive effect may be noticed.

WHEN DO I SEEK PROFESSIONAL HELP?

The Matrix Repatterning Program does not replace the need for professional health care. It is important to remember that, if symptoms persist or become worse, you should consult a health-care professional for more extensive investigation and treatment. If your pain or limitation persists or worsens even after following the procedures outlined below and repeating the process on three or more occasions, it is recommended that you seek professional assistance. A fully comprehensive treatment program would, by necessity, require a significant background in anatomy, physiology, and diagnosis. Certified Matrix Repatterning practitioners are highly trained health professionals able to assess your condition thoroughly and determine whether or not you are a candidate for Matrix Repatterning therapy. They are also able to determine when you might require a referral to another medical specialty. For information on how to locate a Certified Matrix Repatterning Practitioner in your area, please refer to appendix 3.

THE POWER AT OUR FINGERTIPS

Have you ever noticed what happens when you injure yourself? Most people respond to a bump, blow, or strain by reaching for the area with their hands. Somehow, we know intuitively that this will provide some relief. Most of us would assume this is, at most, a form of psychological support or perhaps a placebo (something with no clinical remedial properties that nonetheless tends to soothe). However, as you read below, you will come to understand that this natural tendency is likely a built-in response that may actually serve to realign the normal, healthy integrity of the electromagnetic balance within the body.

Any therapy, in order to be effective, must address the effects of the injury on the molecular structure of the body—the tensegrity matrix. Many therapies influence the electronic or the mechanical properties of the matrix or both. One therapy you may have heard of is trigger point therapy. This technique uses direct pressure on areas within the muscles or *fascia* (the sheets of fibrous tissue in the body) to stimulate tender or *trigger* points. The theory is that this stimulation creates a local physical response (in the muscles) and perhaps a neurological response (in the nervous system) to release the local tension, which is theorized to be the cause of the pain. This and many other approaches are focused on the area of pain, which may or may not be the underlying source of the problem. This is why the same sore spots and pain reoccur and may have to be treated repeatedly.

Matrix Repatterning differs from most other therapies in that it utilizes a process to precisely locate the area of primary involvement, as distinct from any particular area of pain. As previously mentioned, these primary restrictions may have ceased to be actively painful (though they will still be tender to the touch) due to the adaptive tendency of the brain and nervous system. Treatments applied to areas of pain may have temporary benefits and may occasionally effect a more permanent correction. But since they are dependent on the subjective symptom of pain, they may miss the more primary source of the tension pattern, which may in fact be painless.

From your assessment, you may have found certain areas of exquisite tenderness, usually near the center of the primary restrictions. However, as opposed to treatments that require you to goad or rub on these sore spots, we have found that it is possible to restore a normal pattern of tension with Matrix Repatterning without the painful process of stimulating the area of tenderness.

The primary restriction creates an *electronic* change within the tissues. Therefore, a normalizing electrical field may be highly effective in influencing it to return to normal. Remember what I mentioned about our natural tendency to put our hand over an area of injury? We now know that this is a very effective way of superimposing a normal electrical field over an abnormal one. This appears be the basis of the success of many forms of treatment such as Therapeutic Touch, that involve the laying on of hands (Seto et al. 1992). The key, however, to effective and long-lasting pain relief and the restoration of normal tissue function is the ability to precisely locate the areas of primary restriction within the matrix.

In the self-assessment section of this book, you learned how to locate the areas of primary involvement. You discovered for yourself the amazing properties of the matrix, which guided you directly to the source of the problem. You will also discover that, when these primary restrictions are treated, the problem will tend to be significantly improved. After all, the goal of this book is not to keep you focused on problems with the need for repeated and ongoing treatment. We know you have more important things to do in your life—like having fun!

One of the basic principles of Matrix Repatterning is that normal tissue and abnormal tissue have different electromagnetic fields. This is simply the result of the particular arrangement of atoms within each molecule and the amount of energy stored within them. This is something like the difference between the frequency of transmission of one radio station and another station. An area of injury is sending out one particular frequency. This is not the same as the normal, healthy frequency. Assuming your hand is uninjured (please see below under "Forearm, Wrist, and Hand Treatment" if it is), it will broadcast a normal electrical field or frequency. It appears that the hand is particularly suited to provide a more powerful energy signal than other areas of the body (Oschman 2000).

THE KARATE KID

In the movie *The Karate Kid*, the karate master, played by Pat Morita, rubs his hands together vigorously and applies them, with an attendant clap of thunder from the sound effects team, to the injured leg of the

The primary restriction creates an electronic change within the tissues. Therefore, a normalizing electrical field may be highly effective in influencing it to return to normal.

hero of the film. Within minutes, the previously injured limb is ready for action, apparently without much in the way of ill effects.

This example illustrates, albeit in terms of Hollywood's world of fantasy, our inherent understanding that it is possible to effect powerful cures simply by applying our hands to the injured area. In fact, this example, according to a growing body of research, is not that far removed from the truth (Oschman 2000). The powerful sound effects and musical score in the movie underscore the intrinsic electrical power we are actually capable of channeling through our own hands. Various studies have demonstrated an increase in the electrical field generated by the hands of healers (Oshman 2000). The only difference between a healer and you is your intention. With your intention to provide yourself with healing assistance, it has been demonstrated that your electrical field is altered. Trained healers have practiced this more than you may have, but there is really no difference once you have made the decision to enter into a healing relationship with your body.

THE POWER OF THE MIND

Intention and focus appear to play a significant role in the healing process. The electrical fields generated by the body are actually measurable by conventional instruments (Oschmnan 2000), and many studies have confirmed that our thoughts have a powerful influence on many aspects of our health (Sarno 1991; Pert 1997). So, it would follow that your state of mind may also be an import factor as you attempt to provide a form of therapy to assist your body toward health.

Thoughts create electrical energy in the form of nerve impulses, which in turn may be channeled through your hands to your own body. This may be due to the high concentration of nerve endings in the hand. Experience has shown that the best results are obtained when the person applying the treatment—you, in this case—is in a relaxed and peaceful state. While you are performing the treatment it may be helpful to focus gently on a positive image or memory, or simply be in a pleasant environment with a soothing piece of music playing in the background. The positive mental focus could be on something you enjoy doing, the memory of a joyful event or experience, or a place, such as a favorite vacation spot or a room in your house that you enjoy. It would also be helpful to keep your focus on good health and vitality rather than worrying or focusing on the area being damaged in any way. The most important thing is to keep your mind peaceful and relaxed. It has been my experience that anyone can learn to use his or her hands—and mind—in this manner.

ELECTRICAL TREATMENT: SOOTHING IT AWAY

When your hand is placed near the injured area, it appears to tend to influence the electrical field within the molecules in the injured area toward normal. This may be due to the actual arrangement of those molecules being shifted toward normal. This may be why the indicator softens when you locate a primary restriction. It will soften even more significantly as the treatment proceeds, which may indicate that more of the molecules in the injured area are being fully restored to their normal healthy pattern (see figure 5-1).

The entire hand is a potentially powerful healing tool (Seto et al. 1992; Zimmerman 1990); however, the center of the palm of the hand appears to be the most electrically active (figure 5-2).

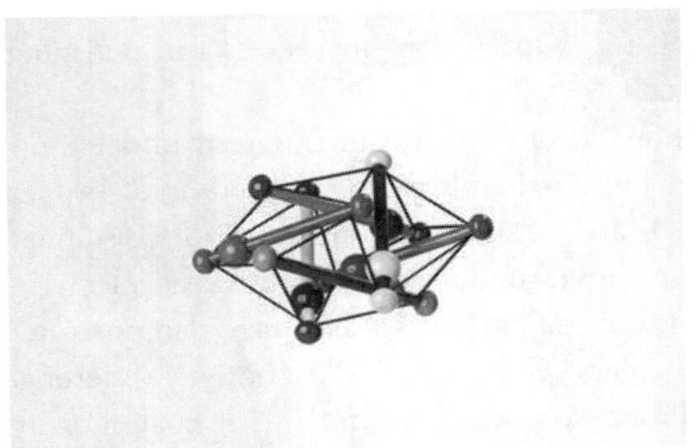

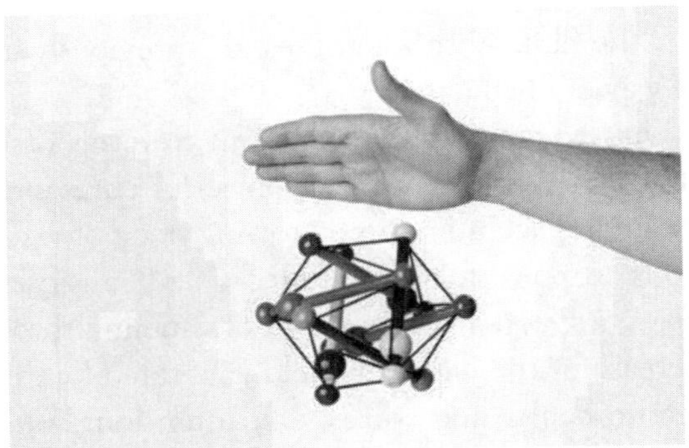

Figure 5-1: Abnormal pattern normalized by placing the hand over the area

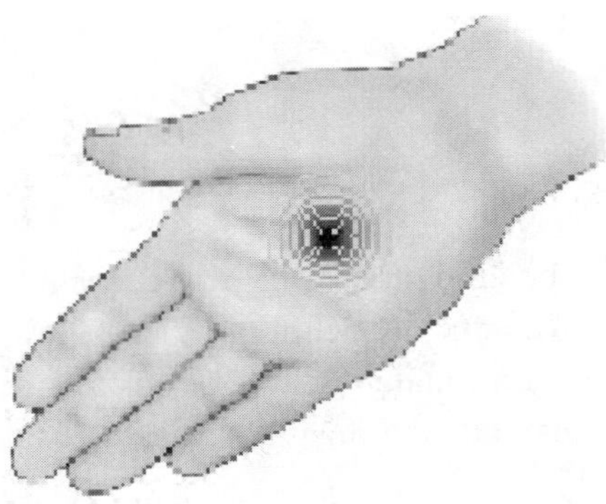

Figure 5-2: Center of electrical field of hand

THE HEALING RESPONSE: THE RELEASE

As you place your hand (especially the palm) over the primary restriction, you may notice that there is a feeling of warmth or *electricity*, both in the area being treated and in your hand as well. This sensation may be associated with what Oschman (2000) refers to as *entrainment*. This is the process whereby one electrical field influences another, causing it to eventually synchronize with the stronger field. In this case, your hand, especially with your conscious intention to direct healing energy to the affected area, will create a strong field relative to the injured site. The feeling may be created by the actual realignment of the molecules in the primary restriction as electrical energy is literally released from the molecular bonds. It has also been proposed that this process may actually facilitate the conversion of the cellular matrix from a solid (gel) state to a more liquid (sol) state (Marsland 1942). More recent evidence of the role of water in the structure of the cellular matrix is described by Pollack (2001) and Tanaka (1981). If you don't feel the energy sensation, don't worry. With time and practice you may find that this awareness will become heightened.

You may become aware of several other changes as you proceed with treatment. One is a change in your breathing. You may find that your breathing becomes more relaxed and even. With this change, you may also find that you become more relaxed. You may also notice that your thoughts become clearer and less focused on worry. As you notice each of these changes, simply relax and enjoy them. Just notice how good it feels. It's almost like an all-expense-paid vacation, without having to drive to the airport!

If you are able to feel these sensations, continue to hold your hand over the affected area until you feel a *release.* The release is a deepening of relaxation associated with a balancing of energy within the area being treated. There are several physiological responses that have been found to be associated with this common experience among people engaged in the healing process (Oschman 1994). What you may notice is a sudden increase in the softening of the indicator, as well as the area being treated, along with some of the breathing and relaxation responses mentioned above. These changes herald the completion of the Repatterning process.

At that point, if you wish to, you may scan the area of the original primary restriction, moving in circles around it to scan for another part of the injury. Your indicator will respond to the new location. Simply repeat the process of treatment until you feel another release and/or the indicator softens noticeably. Once you find that the indicator no longer softens in response to any other scanned locations, your treatment is complete.

ELECTRICAL TREATMENT FOR THE WHOLE BODY

In most cases, electrical treatment will be the primary form of self-treatment you will use. This technique should help you address most common day-to-day structural injuries. If you find after two or three sessions that you're unable to correct the problem, you may wish to follow the guidelines for mechanical treatment outlined in the next section. The following pages contain some of the most common treatments for the entire body. The main areas include:

1. Head
2. Teeth
3. Neck
4. Rib cage, including major internal organs
5. Arms and hands
6. Upper back
7. Lower back
8. Hips and pelvis
9. Legs and feet

Step-by-Step Guidelines for Electrical Treatment

Complete the following steps to treat each area of primary restriction. As you proceed, keep in mind these general guidelines: treat the most significant area first; use the Body Scan to determine the next-most-important area requiring treatment and repeat the process; then retest using the Body Check to verify the success of your treatment. Always remember to keep your movements within your comfort level.

1. Make yourself as comfortable as possible, sitting or lying down.
2. Place your hand over the center of the area you have determined to be the primary restriction using the Body Scan (chapter 4).

3. Monitor the amount of tension or resistance in the indicator (thigh muscle or joints of the hand). The primary restriction will also soften as the treatment proceeds.
4. Feel for softening of the indicator and/or the primary restriction as you fine-tune your position over the treatment area. You may place one or both hands over the primary restriction or keep one hand on the indicator during treatment.
5. Relax and breathe fully during the treatment and consciously relax the area being treated.
6. Be aware of the treatment site. As the treatment is nearing its conclusion, you may notice that the indicator and the treatment site will suddenly both become much softer. This is referred to as a release. This process may take from one to ten minutes.
7. The treatment may need to be repeated several times over one to three days. This can be done while you're watching a TV show, while reading, or even while riding in a car (not recommended if you are the driver!).
8. For primary restrictions located in the upper back or the back of the rib cage, you may wish to enlist the assistance of a family member or a friend who can place their hands over the appropriate sites. You will be able to guide them by monitoring the indicator as they move their hands over the target area.

ELECTRICAL SELF-TREATMENT

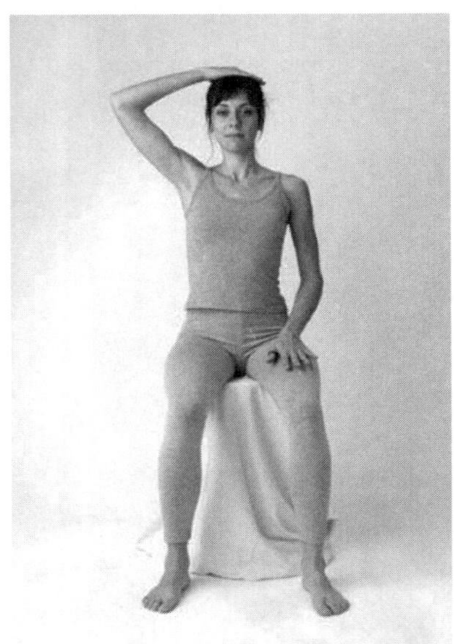

Top of head: Place hand over the primary restriction. Monitor using an indicator on thigh. Gently move the hand to increase the softening of the indicator. Maintain the contact until you feel a significant softening of the indicator.

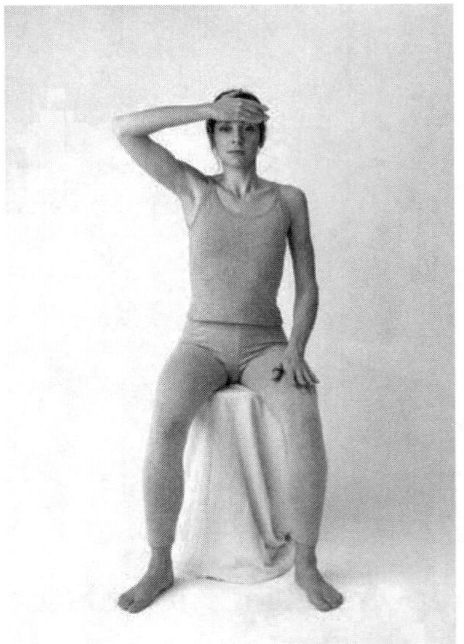

Forehead: Place hand over the primary restriction. Monitor using an indicator on thigh. Gently move the hand to increase the softening of the indicator. Maintain the contact until you feel a significant softening of the indicator.

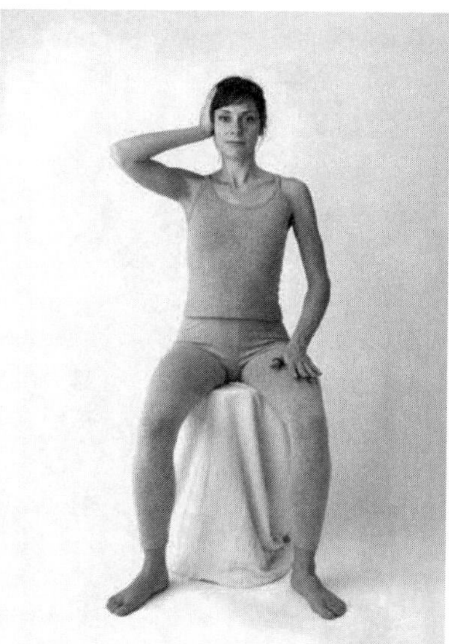

Side of head: Place hand over the primary restriction. Monitor using an indicator on thigh. Gently move the hand to increase the softening of the indicator. Maintain the contact until you feel a significant softening of the indicator.

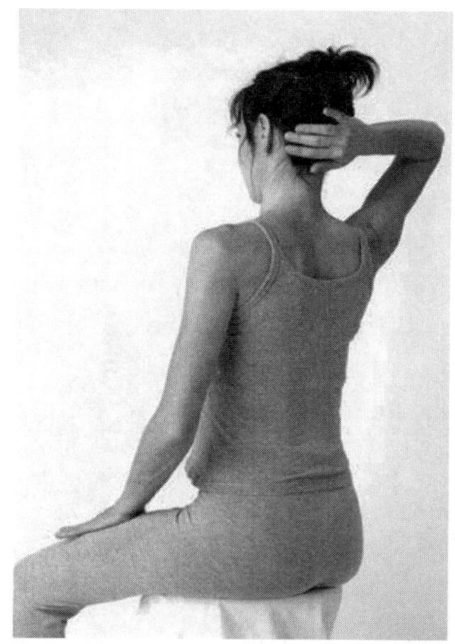

Back of head: Place hand over the primary restriction. Monitor using an indicator on thigh. Gently move the hand to increase the softening of the indicator. Maintain the contact until you feel a significant softening of the indicator.

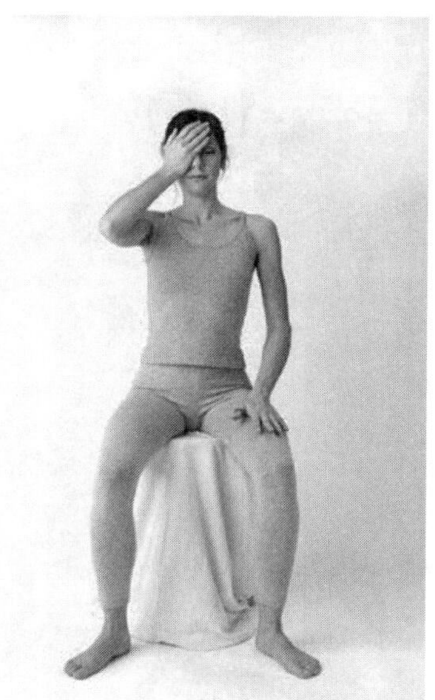

Eyes: Place hand over the primary restriction. Monitor using an indicator. Gently move the hand to increase the softening of the indicator. Maintain the contact until you feel a significant softening of the indicator.

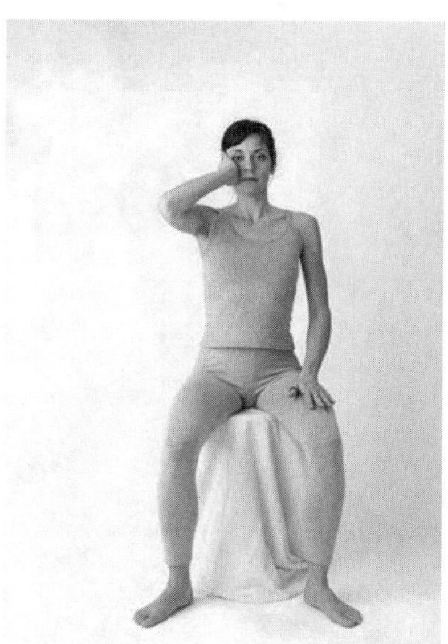

Cheekbone: Place hand over the primary restriction. Monitor using an indicator. Gently move the hand to increase the softening of the indicator. Maintain the contact until you feel a significant softening of the indicator.

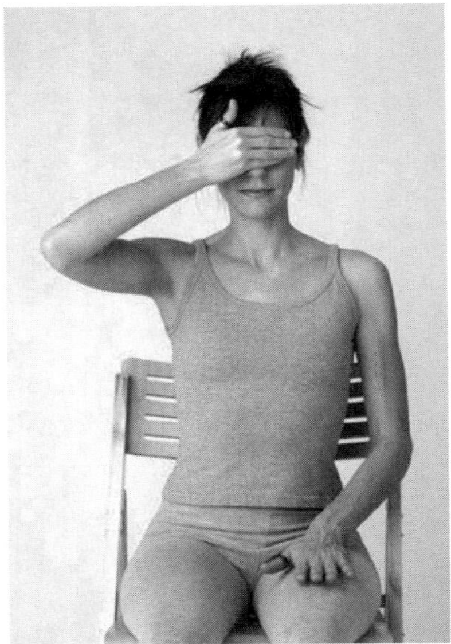

Nose: Place hand over the primary restriction. Monitor using an indicator. Gently move the hand to increase the softening of the indicator. Maintain the contact until you feel a significant softening of the indicator.

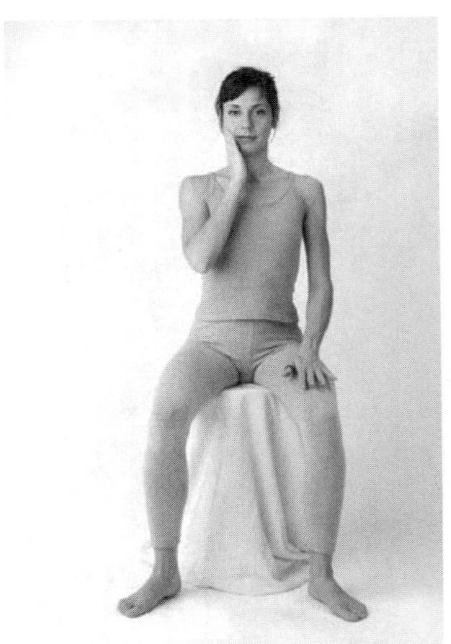

Jaws: Place hand over the primary restriction. Monitor using an indicator. Gently move the hand to increase the softening of the indicator. Maintain the contact until you feel a significant softening of the indicator.

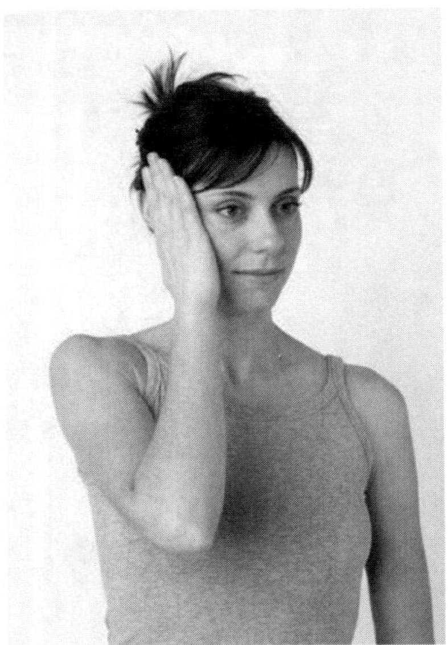

Teeth (upper and lower): Place hand over the primary restriction. Monitor using an indicator. Gently move the hand to increase the softening of the indicator. Maintain the contact until you feel a significant softening of the indicator.

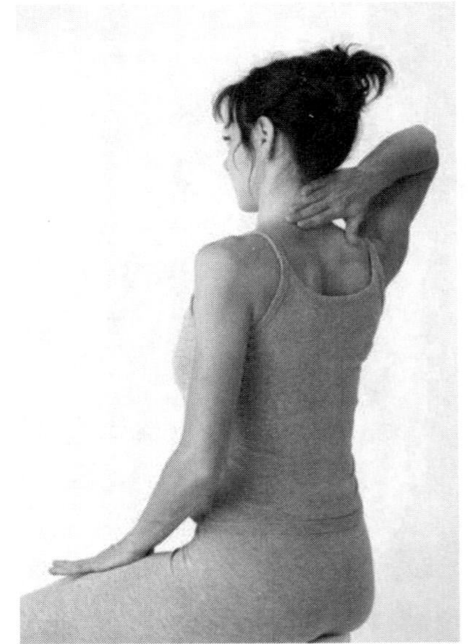

Lower neck: Place hand over the primary restriction. Monitor using an indicator. Gently move the hand to increase the softening of the indicator. Maintain the contact until you feel a significant softening of the indicator.

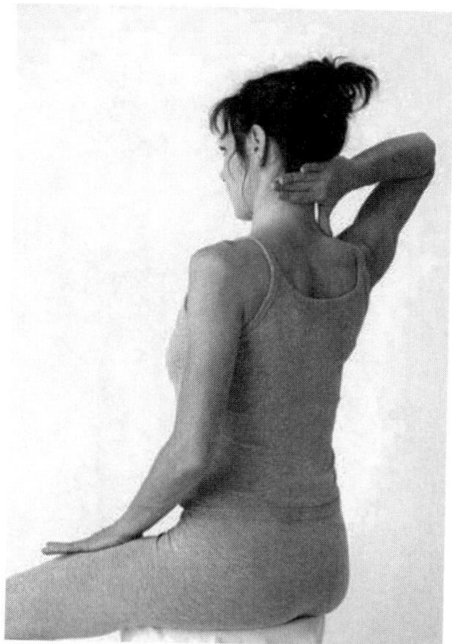

Upper neck: Place hand over the primary restriction. Monitor using an indicator. Gently move the hand to increase the softening of the indicator. Maintain the contact until you feel a significant softening of the indicator.

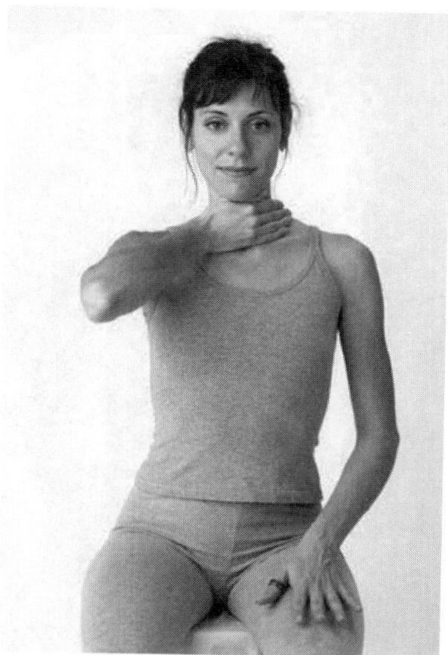

Throat: Place hand over the primary restriction. Monitor using an indicator. Gently move the hand to increase the softening of the indicator. Maintain the contact until you feel a significant softening of the indicator.

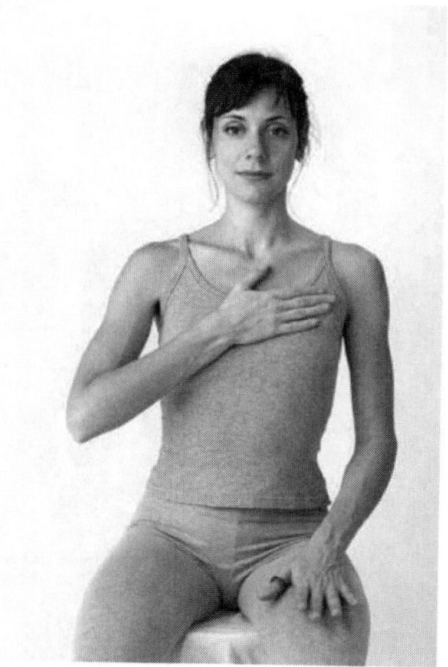

Front of chest, upper: Place hand over the primary restriction. Monitor using an indicator. Gently move the hand to increase the softening of the indicator. Maintain the contact until you feel a significant softening of the indicator.

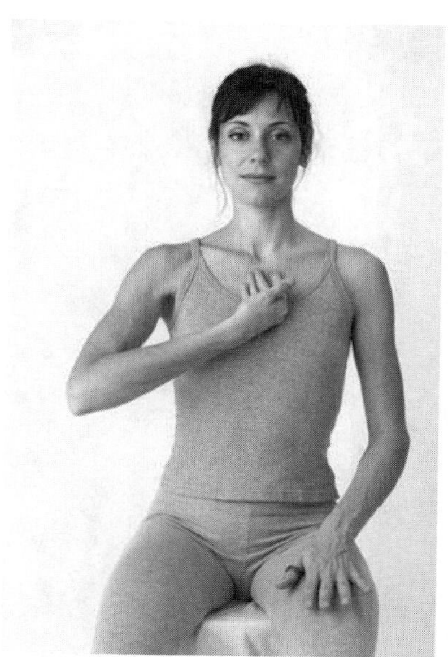

Back of chest, upper back: Place hand over the primary restriction. Monitor using an indicator. Gently move the hand to increase the softening of the indicator. Maintain the contact until you feel a significant softening of the indicator.

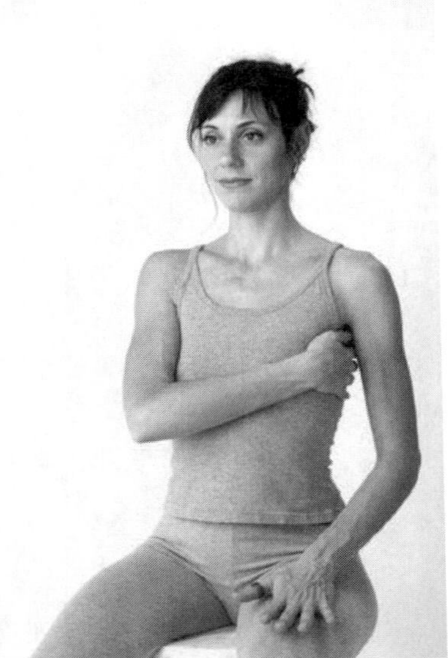

Side of upper chest: Place hand over the primary restriction. Monitor using an indicator. Gently move the hand to increase the softening of the indicator. Maintain the contact until you feel a significant softening of the indicator.

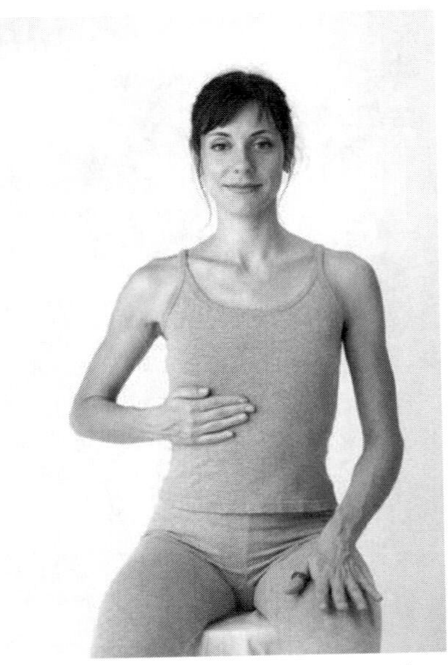

Front of lower chest: Place hand over the primary restriction. Monitor using an indicator. Gently move the hand to increase the softening of the indicator. Maintain the contact until you feel a significant softening of the indicator.

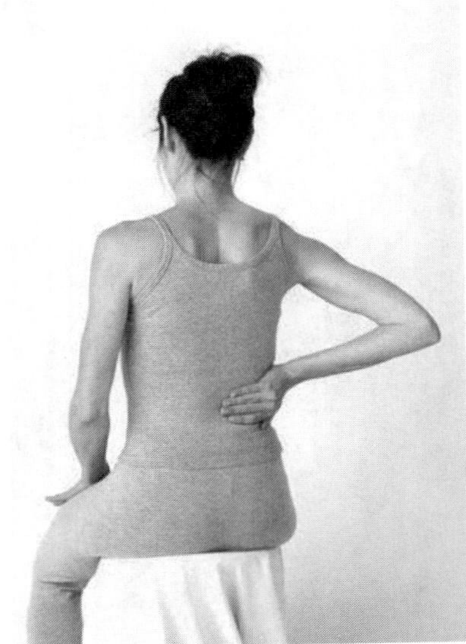

Back of lower chest: Place hand over the primary restriction. Monitor using an indicator. Gently move the hand to increase the softening of the indicator. Maintain the contact until you feel a significant softening of the indicator.

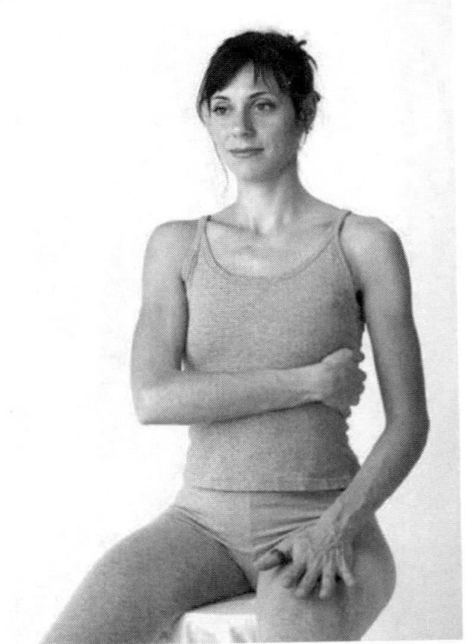

Side of lower chest: Place hand over the primary restriction. Monitor using an indicator. Gently move the hand to increase the softening of the indicator. Maintain the contact until you feel a significant softening of the indicator.

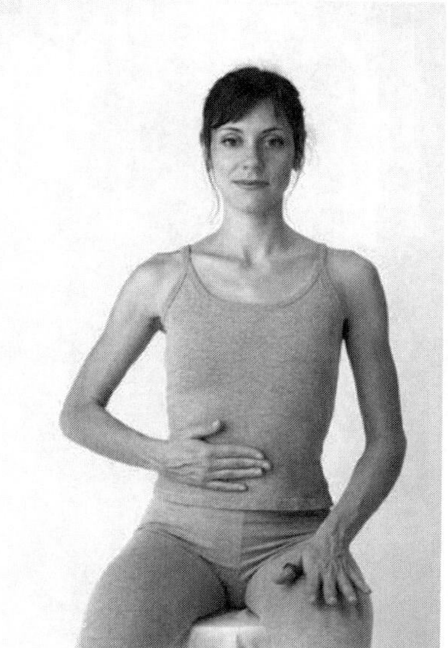

Upper abdomen (side): Place hand over the primary restriction. Monitor using an indicator. Gently move the hand to increase the softening of the indicator. Maintain the contact until you feel a significant softening of the indicator.

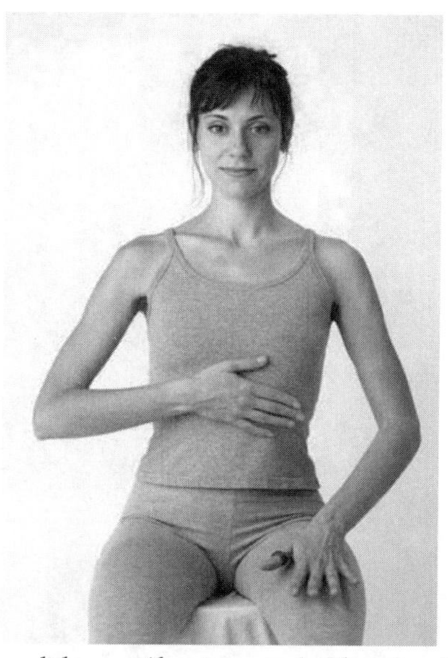

Upper abdomen (front, center): Place hand over the primary restriction. Monitor using an indicator. Gently move the hand to increase the softening of the indicator. Maintain the contact until you feel a significant softening of the indicator.

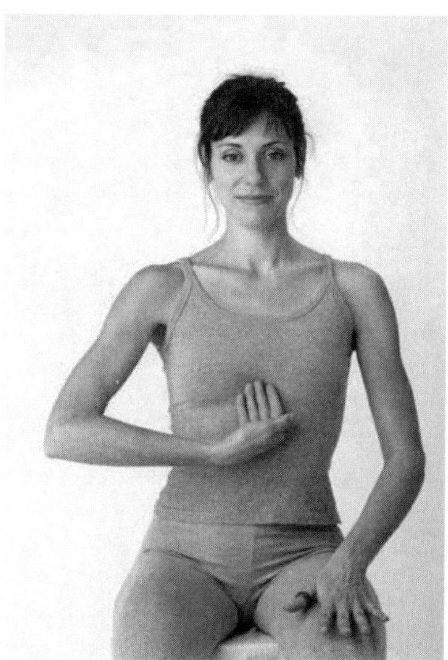

Upper abdomen (back, center): Place hand over the primary restriction. Monitor using an indicator. Gently move the hand to increase the softening of the indicator. Maintain the contact until you feel a significant softening of the indicator.

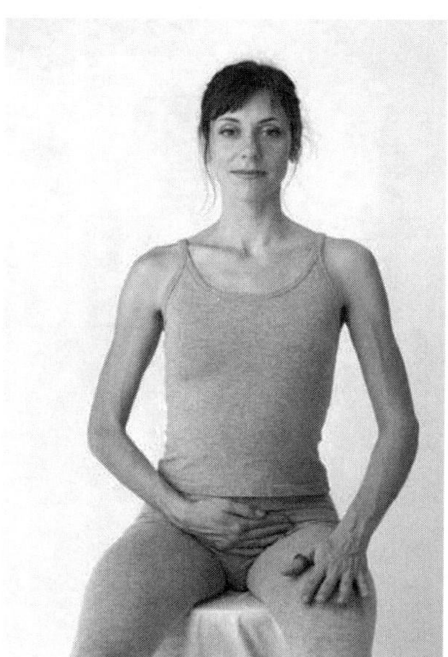

Pelvis, lower abdomen (front): Place hand over the primary restriction. Monitor using an indicator. Gently move the hand to increase the softening of the indicator. Maintain the contact until you feel a significant softening of the indicator.

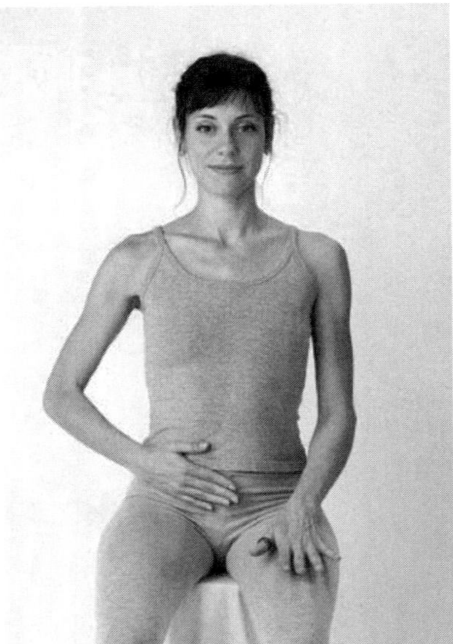

Pelvis, lower abdomen (front, side): Place hand over the primary restriction. Monitor using an indicator. Gently move the hand to increase the softening of the indicator. Maintain the contact until you feel a significant softening of the indicator.

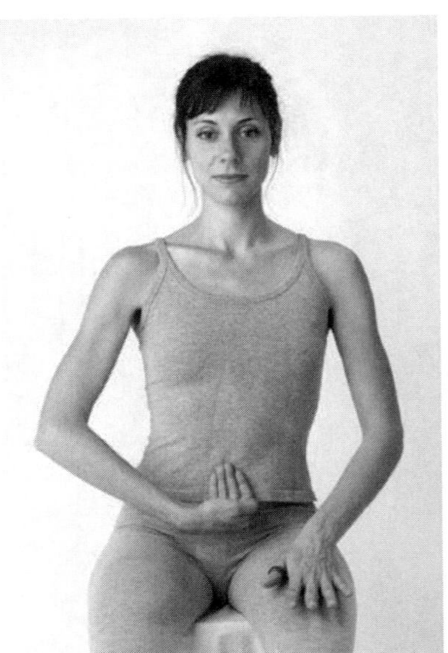

Pelvis (side): Place hand over the primary restriction. Monitor using an indicator. Gently move the hand to increase the softening of the indicator. Maintain the contact until you feel a significant softening of the indicator.

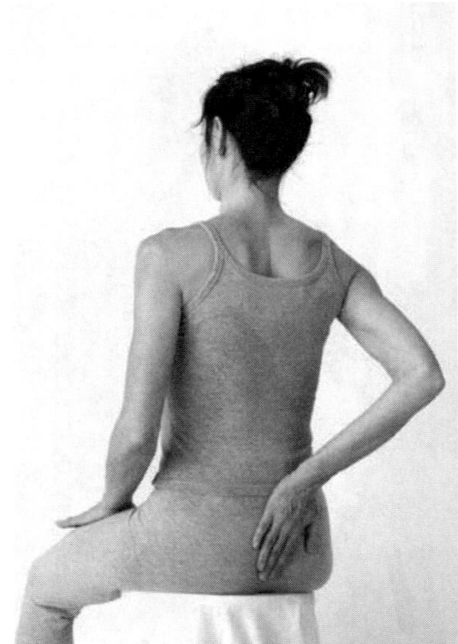

Pelvis (back): Place hand over the primary restriction. Monitor using an indicator. Gently move the hand to increase the softening of the indicator. Maintain the contact until you feel a significant softening of the indicator.

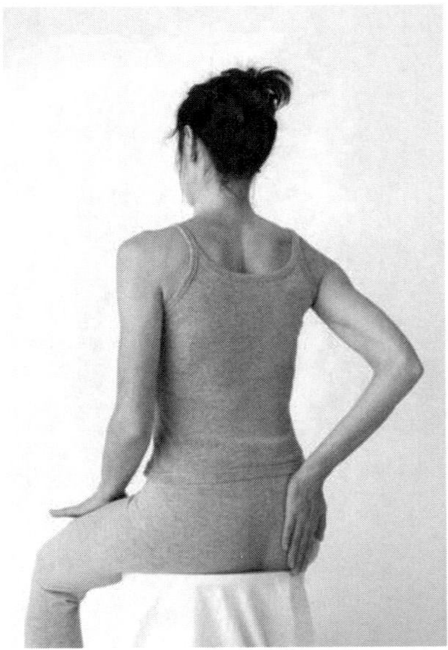

Pelvis (back, side): Place hand over the primary restriction. Monitor using an indicator. Gently move the hand to increase the softening of the indicator. Maintain the contact until you feel a significant softening of the indicator.

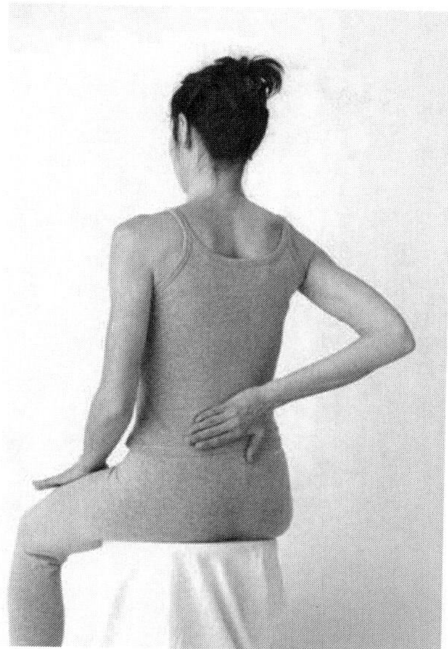

Low back: Place hand over the primary restriction. Monitor using an indicator. Gently move the hand to increase the softening of the indicator. Maintain the contact until you feel a significant softening of the indicator.

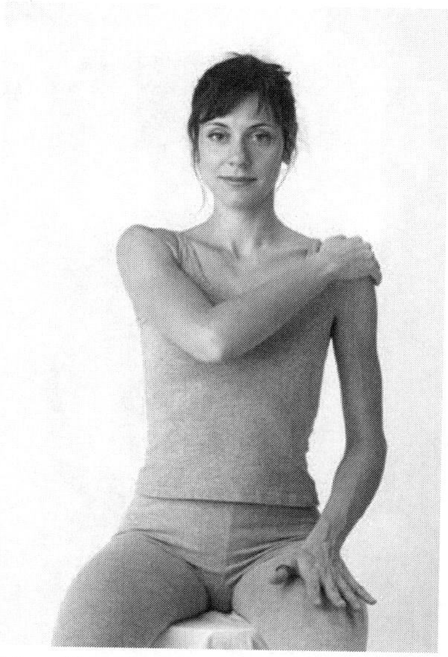

Shoulder: Place hand over the primary restriction. Monitor using an indicator. Gently move the hand to increase the softening of the indicator. Maintain the contact until you feel a significant softening of the indicator.

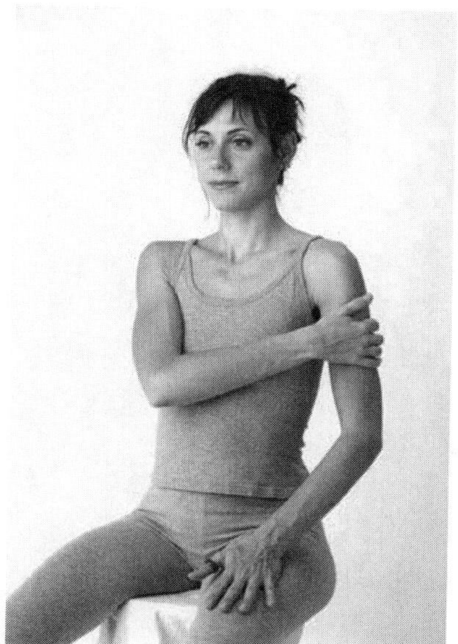

Upper arm: Place hand over the primary restriction. Monitor using an indicator. Gently move the hand to increase the softening of the indicator. Maintain the contact until you feel a significant softening of the indicator.

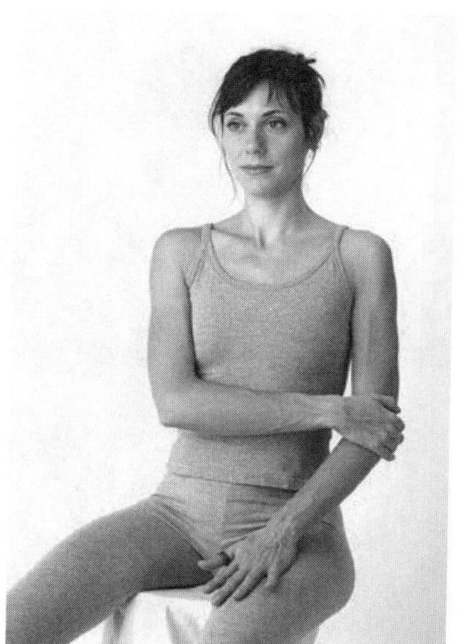

Elbow: Place hand over the primary restriction. Monitor using an indicator. Gently move the hand to increase the softening of the indicator. Maintain the contact until you feel a significant softening of the indicator.

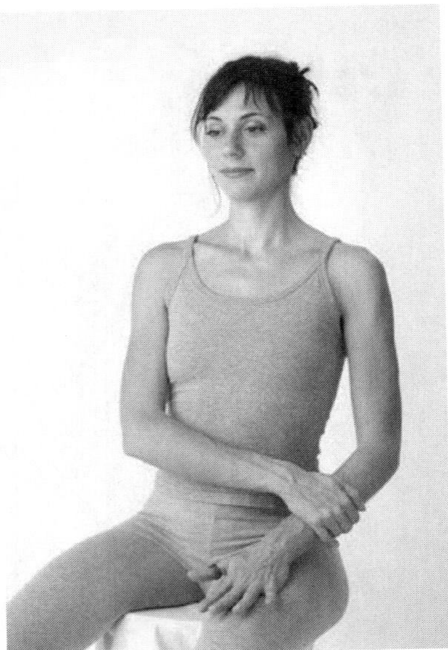

Forearm: Place hand over the primary restriction. Monitor using an indicator. Gently move the hand to increase the softening of the indicator. Maintain the contact until you feel a significant softening of the indicator.

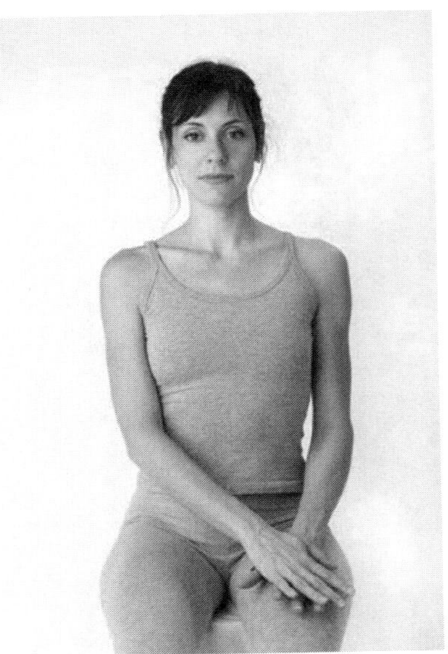

Hand: Place hand over the primary restriction. Monitor using an indicator. Gently move the hand to increase the softening of the indicator. Maintain the contact until you feel a significant softening of the indicator.

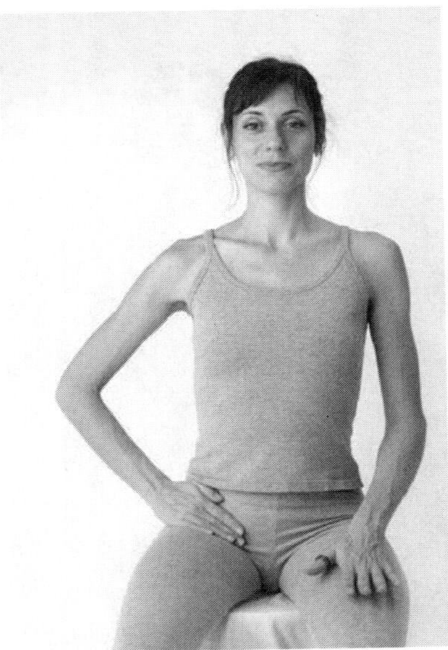

Hip: Place hand over the primary restriction. Monitor using an indicator. Gently move the hand to increase the softening of the indicator. Maintain the contact until you feel a significant softening of the indicator.

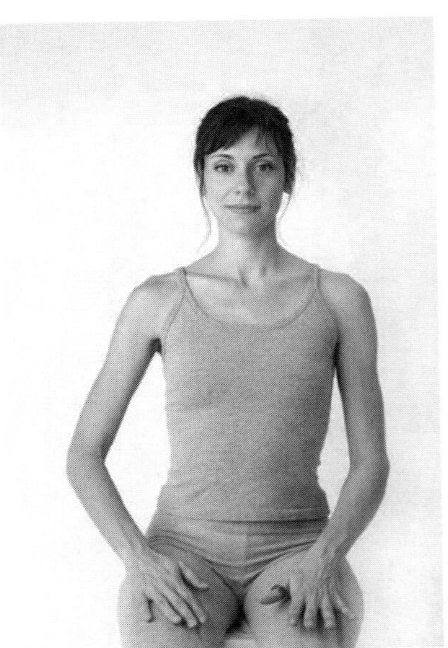

Thigh: Place hand over the primary restriction. Monitor using an indicator (left thigh in this example). Gently move the hand to increase the softening of the indicator. Maintain the contact until you feel a significant softening of the indicator.

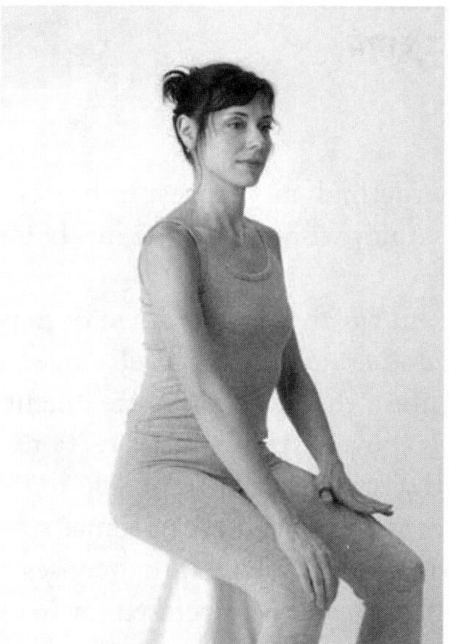

Knee: Place hand over the primary restriction. Monitor using an indicator on the other thigh. Gently move the hand to increase the softening of the indicator. Maintain the contact until you feel a significant softening of the indicator.

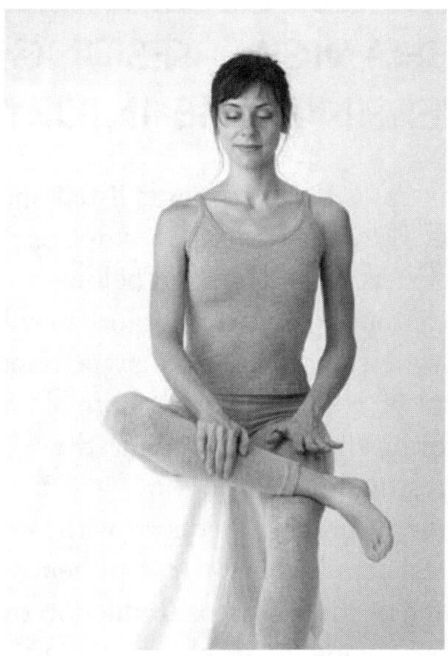

Lower leg: Place hand over the primary restriction. Monitor using an indicator on the other thigh. Gently move the hand to increase the softening of the indicator. Maintain the contact until you feel a significant softening of the indicator.

SCAR TISSUE ISSUES

Scar tissue will often be revealed as a primary restriction through the Body Scan. Once you have determined that it's a priority through your self-assessment, you may treat it using the following method:

1. Place the center of the palm of your hand over the most reactive area, based on the reaction of your indicator. Superficial surgical scars are often less important from a structural perspective. They may, however, give you a clue as to the location of the more significant scar tissue deeper within your body. The deeper scars are often the ones that require treatment. The indicator is the most reliable way to locate the true source of the primary restriction. Use it to guide you in determining where to place your treating hand. Other sources of scar tissue may not be evident from the surface. These may include remnants of old infections or inflammatory conditions. If you are aware of any of these types of conditions, you can simply scan the area to precisely locate the presence of any scar tissue in the area.
2. Once you have found the location of the most significant occurrence of the scar tissue, simply place the center of one of your hands over the area while using the other hand to monitor the indicator. Next, gently push your hand into the area until you find the depth where the indicator becomes the softest. This will provide you with information about the depth of the scar tissue and allow you to access it for treatment more efficiently.
3. Continue to keep your treating hand in place until you feel a release in the area of treatment or you feel an increase in softening of the indicator.

Because scar tissue may never fully return to its normal state, it is recommended that you check it from time to time and treat it on a regular basis. This will often maintain it in a relatively flexible state and reduce the chances of it creating strain elsewhere in the body.

MECHANICAL TESTING AND TREATMENT: REVERSING THE INJURY

In most cases the treatments listed above should resolve most structural imbalances. If, however, the area you have already treated does not respond after 2-3 sessions, you may wish to add the mechanical component of treatment described below.

Certain aspects of an injury may be related to the direction in which it was strained or impacted. The effectiveness of treatment may be improved by finding out which *direction* the molecules need to move in order to be restored to their normal balanced state. You can confirm the direction of treatment needed by monitoring the indicator while the area of primary restriction is moved in different directions. If the primary restriction is in a bone, it can be pulled or pushed lengthwise, squeezed from side-to-side, bent or twisted in different directions with one hand while the indicator is monitored for maximal softening. You can also actively move the joint being treated in different directions. The direction that causes the greatest softening of the indicator (reduction of the resistance barrier) is the direction to be used for treatment.

For example, stubbing your toe involves a compression of the bones and joints of the foot (see figure 5-3 below).

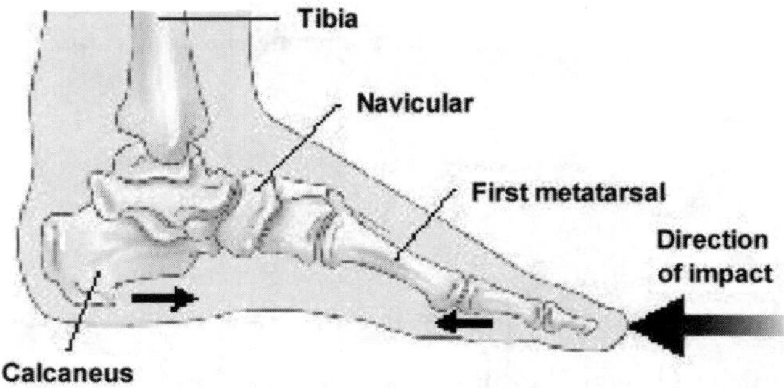

Figure 5-3: Stubbing your toe

With this type of injury, the bones and/or the joints of the foot will be compressed from front to back due to the fact that the molecules got pushed together by the injury. Part of your treatment could include a stretching of the toe by grabbing onto the end of it and pulling it lengthwise (See Figure 5-4 below).

This type of treatment requires only a very gentle force, as your purpose is to simply release the energy trapped in the molecules. The amount of force is just enough to feel a slight pressure in the area being treated (see The Resistance Barrier, above). It should always feel comfortable, and often it will feel pleasant, as the energy in the molecules is released. At a certain point you will feel a similar *release* sensation as you would for the electrical treatment, in the area being treated. This is often accompanied by a relaxation of the joints and muscles and a feeling of warmth or tingling. While monitoring the indicator during treatment, you will notice that it will also relax significantly when the full release has been achieved.

Treating Bones

If you are aware, for example, that your injury happened when you fell directly onto your knee, the indicator will confirm this by increasing in softening when you pull on the thigh lengthwise from the knee. Remember, bone is remarkably plastic, in spite of its apparent hardness and rigidity (Duncan 1995). There may also be an expansion of the end of the thigh (near the knee), due to the apparent distortion of the bone and surrounding structures away from the center of impact. In general, impact appears to cause the molecules near the point of impact to spread radially (away from the center of impact), thus causing an apparent widening of the end of the bone. The indicator will soften when you compress this area in toward the center.

The molecules within the shaft of the bone also appear to be compressed or shortened in the direction of the impact. Other bone injuries may involve stretching, bending, or twisting. These types of injuries may occur with various types of strains or impact injuries. For example, ankle sprains may cause a bowing of the long bones of the lower leg as well as restrictions within the joints.

Figure 5-4: Reversing a stubbed toe

Mechanical Treatment of Bones

Use one hand to test the indicator. You may need to use the finger or thumb pull indicator for joints in the upper limb. Scan with the other hand to determine that the bone is the primary restriction to be treated.

With the scanning hand, grasp the end of the bone that is farthest away from the body (for example, for the leg, grasp it just above the ankle). Test the direction of the primary restriction by stressing it in each of the directions illustrated below. Fine-tune the position back and forth to maximize the softening of the indicator. The ends of the bones should also be tested for expansion by squeezing them in from the sides.

Find a comfortable position to support and maintain this direction until you feel a release in the area being treated and/or in the indicator.

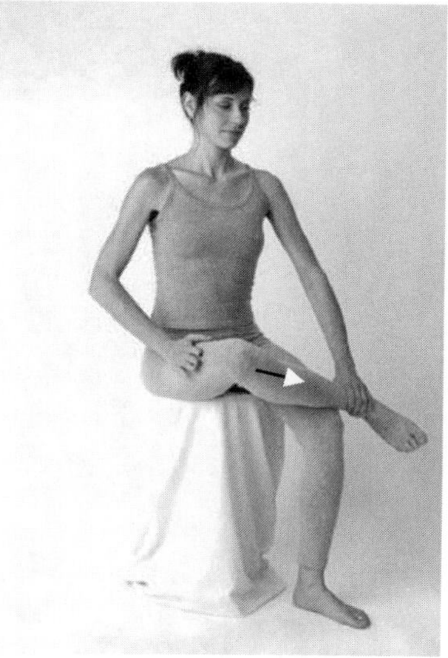

Lengthwise compression test/treatment: The bone or joint has been compressed. Test by grasping the end of the bone and pulling it lengthwise. Softening of the indicator verifies this as the direction of treatment.

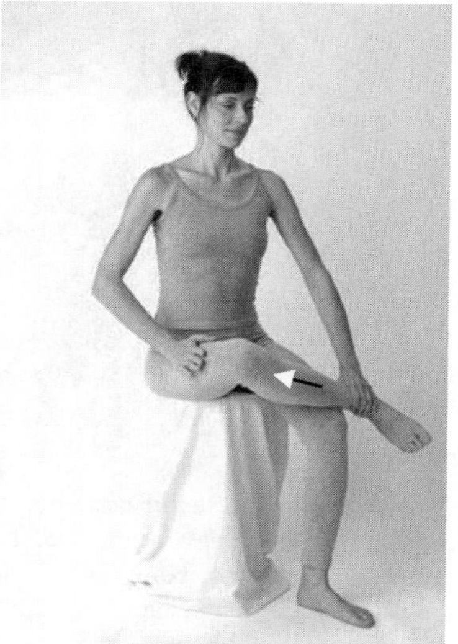

Lengthwise stretching test/treatment: The bone or joint has been stretched. Test by pushing toward the joint. Softening of the indicator verifies this as the direction of treatment.

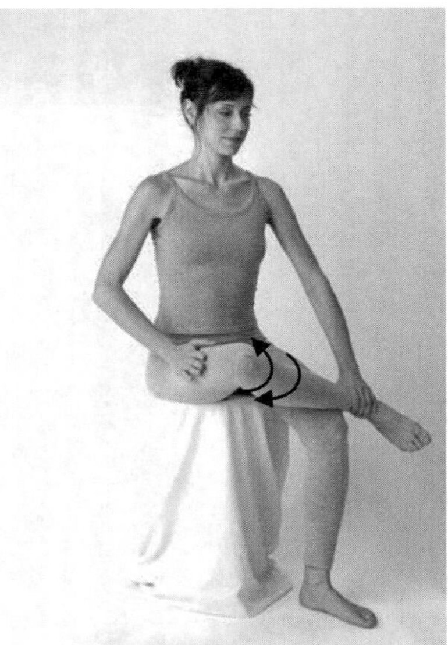

Twisting test/treatment: The bone or joint has been twisted. Test by grasping the bone and twisting it in both directions. Softening of the indicator verifies the direction of treatment.

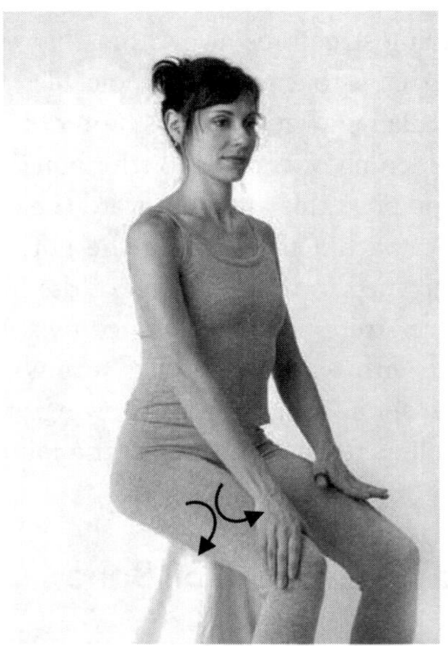

Bowing test/treatment: The bone has been bowed sideways or front to back. Test by grasping one end of the bone and bowing it from side to side or forward and backward. Softening of the indicator verifies the direction of treatment.

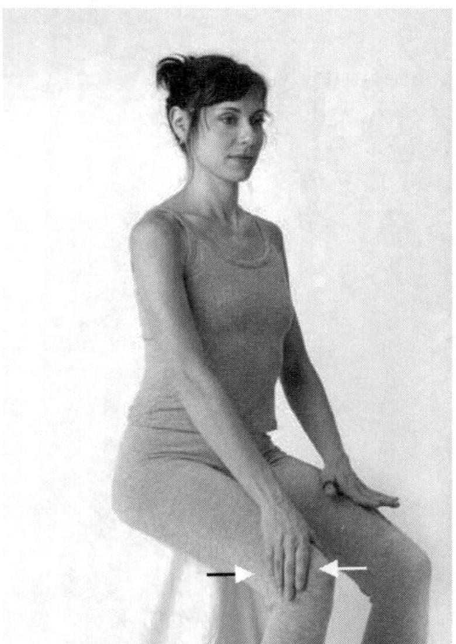

Long bone expansion test/treatment: The ends of the bone have expanded. Test by squeezing the end of the bone toward the center as you would squeeze a piece of fruit. Softening of the indicator verifies this as the direction of treatment.

Joints: Where One Bonehead Meets Another

Joints are where two or more bones join together. Joints are composed of fibrous tissue and other relatively flexible components. They tend to absorb less of the energy of an injury than the dense bones on either side of them. Joints can, however, form an important part of a persistent injury and, as such, may need to be addressed separately. Once a primary area has been identified, it is possible to differentiate between the bone and the joint by simply moving the scanning hand to center over the bones or the joint between two bones. A primary restriction in a joint will be a small area between the bones as determined by the indicator. The tenderness will also be located directly over this area. For spinal joints, please refer to the section on back pain in chapter 6.

In the case of a primary restriction located within a joint, the direction may be tested by moving it in different directions to see which direction causes the indicator to soften the most.

Joint Direction

Joints have two types of movement, active and passive. *Active movements* (also referred to as *physiological movements*) are movements that you can perform by actively using the muscles that normally move the joint. This includes the movements that would normally be performed in daily activities. For example, at the knee the leg moves like a hinge, backward and forward in relation to the thigh. *Passive movements* (also referred to as *nonphysiological movements* or *joint play*) can only be performed by force exerted outside the actual muscles of the joint. These are typically very slight movements that represent the degree to which the joint can accommodate external forces applied to it. In a sense, this is a protective mechanism to allow the joint to give slightly when overstressed or overloaded. For example, the knee can be moved backward and forward, from side to side, twisted to the right and the left, side bent to the right and the left, pulled away from the thigh and pushed toward the thigh. Treatment of joints may include all of these components

Active Test and Treatment

Use one hand to test the indicator. Scan with the other hand to determine that the joint is the primary restriction to be treated.

While maintaining contact with the indicator with one hand and the primary restriction over the joint with the other, slowly move the joint actively in different directions. Determine which direction causes the greatest softening of the indicator. Move the joint back and forth to fine-tune the position and maximize the softening of the indicator. Find a comfortable position to support this position until you feel a release in the area being treated and/or in the indicator.

Passive Test and Treatment

Use one hand to test the indicator. You may need to use the finger or thumb pull indicator for joints in the upper limb. Scan with the other hand to determine that the joint is the primary restriction to be treated.

With the scanning hand, grasp the bone near the joint that is farthest away from the body (for example, for the elbow, grasp the forearm rather than the upper arm). Move this bone in the directions indicated by the white arrows in the diagrams below.

Fine-tune the position back and forth to maximize the softening of the indicator. Maintain this direction until you feel a release in the area being treated and/or in the indicator. Find a comfortable position to support this position until you feel a release in the area being treated and/or in the indicator.

In each of the diagrams below, the black arrows indicate the direction of the restriction within the joint and the white arrows indicate the direction for testing and treating the joint.

The joint has been compressed. Test by pulling one bone away from the other.

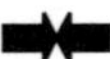

The joint has been stretched apart. Test by pushing one bone toward the other.

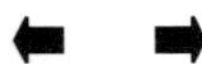

The joint has been bent sideways or backward or forward. Test by bending one bone sideways in one direction and then the other.

The joint has been shifted to one side or backwards or forwards. This is like two blocks that are stacked with one being off center in relation to the other. Test by shifting the bone sideways in both directions.

The joint has been twisted. Test by twisting the bone in both directions.

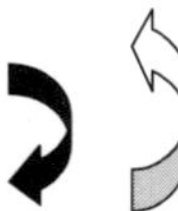

Parts of the body that often include a directional mechanical component include all of the long bones of the body—the toes, the lower legs, the thighs, the fingers, the forearms, and the arms, as well as the joints between these bones and the joints of the spine. You may not always remember how an area may have been injured, but simply testing in each direction can allow you to perform a much more precise and effective treatment.

The test for a mechanical pattern of strain within a part of the body is the response of the indicator to the direction in which it is pushed, pulled, bent, or twisted. The direction that causes the greatest softening of the indicator is the one that will also normalize the primary restriction. Simply maintain this direction or joint position until there is a complete release.

If a pattern of mechanical imbalance is not obvious, simply proceed with the electrical treatment. In most cases this will resolve most of the primary restrictions in the area. The purpose of the mechanical treatment is only to improve the efficiency of the process.

A trained Matrix Repatterning Practitioner will combine several components of treatment, which is often more complete and more rapid in its effect. This is not to say that you cannot help yourself significantly. The self-treatment program outlined in this book is very effective at dealing with most minor complaints and providing relief in many chronic and acute conditions.

For mechanical treatment, never force the movement or position. If pain develops during treatment, slowly return to a comfortable position.

MECHANICAL SELF TREATMENT

You may have performed an electrical treatment from the previous section, and found that you were unable to fully resolve the primary restriction. In this case, you may wish to add the mechanical treatment procedures listed below. In each of these treatments, move the end of the long bone (for bone treatment) furthest away from the center of the body, as indicated by the accompanying photographs, while monitoring the indicator. For active joint treatment, move the joints in the area of primary restriction slightly in different directions with the scanning hand placed over it while monitoring the indicator. For passive joint treatment, grasp the bone near the joint furthest away from the center of the body and move it in the directions described in the preceding section. Maintain the contact and the position until you feel a significant softening of the indicator and/or the primary restriction. **Be sure to move only within your comfortable range.**

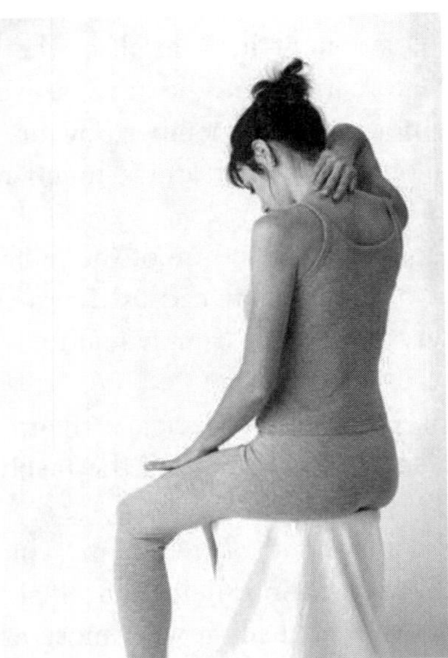

Neck, forward bend: Place hand over primary restriction. Monitor using an indicator. Slowly bend head forward until indicator is maximally softened. Maintain until you feel significant softening of indicator.

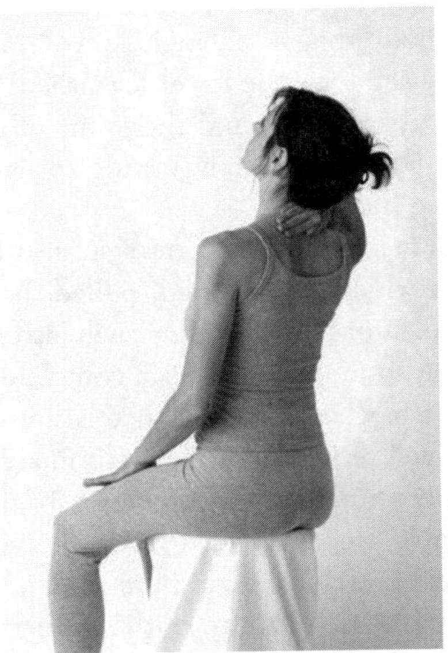

Neck, backward bend: Place hand over primary restriction. Monitor using an indicator. Slowly bend head backward until indicator is maximally softened. Maintain until you feel significant softening of indicator.

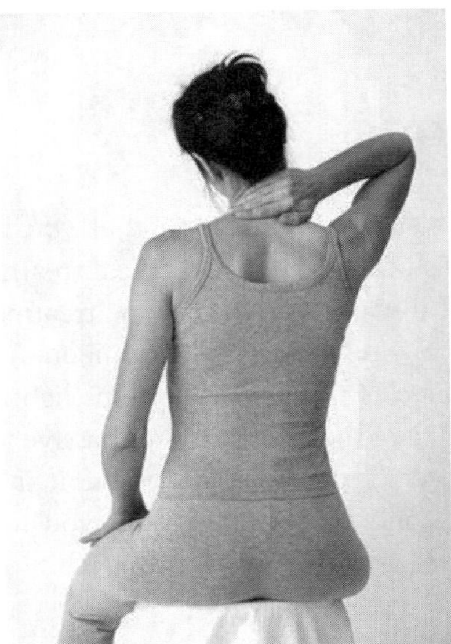

Neck, side bend: Place hand over primary restriction. Monitor using an indicator. Slowly bend head to right or left until indicator is maximally softened. Maintain until you feel significant softening of indicator.

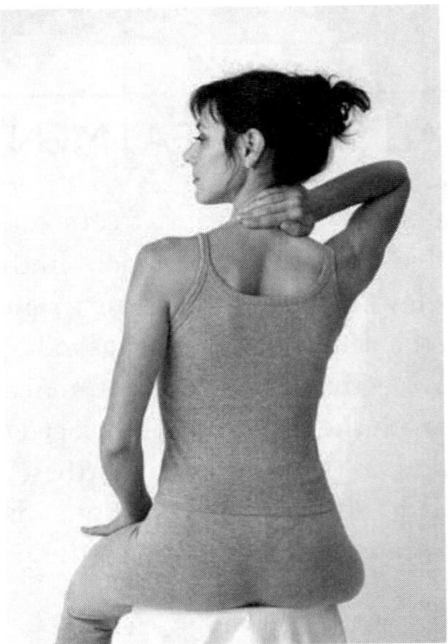

Neck, rotation: Place hand over primary restriction. Monitor using an indicator. Slowly rotate head right or left until indicator is maximally softened. Maintain until you feel significant softening of indicator.

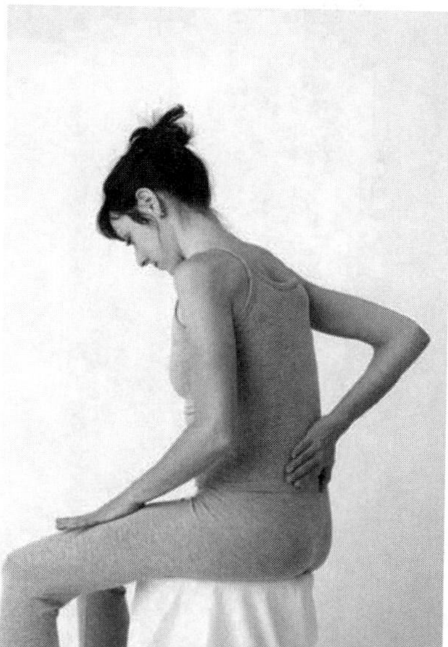

Low back, forward bend: Place hand over primary restriction. Monitor using an indicator. Slowly bend forward at the waist until indicator is maximally softened. Maintain until you feel significant softening of indicator.

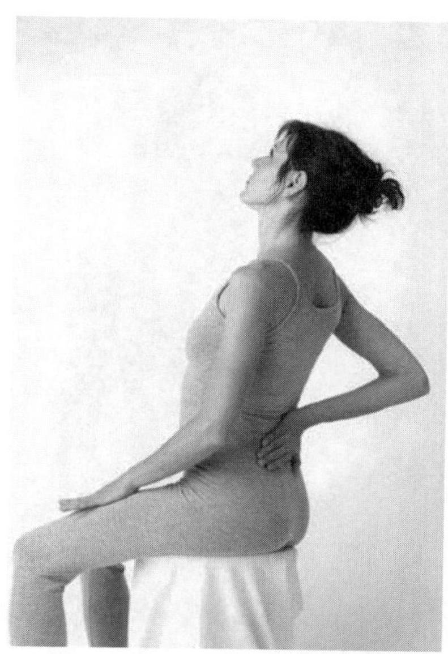

Low back, backward bend: Place hand over primary restriction. Monitor using an indicator. Slowly bend backward waist until indicator is maximally softened. Maintain until you feel significant softening of indicator.

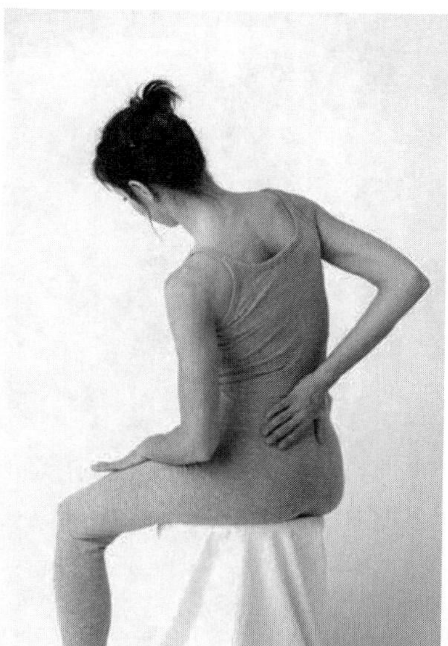

Low back, side bend: Place hand over primary restriction. Monitor using an indicator. Slowly bend at the waist to the right or left until indicator is maximally softened. Maintain until you feel significant softening of indicator.

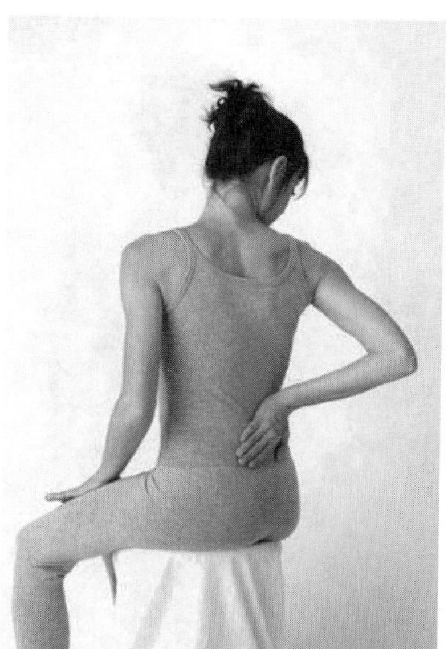

Low back, rotation: Place hand over primary restriction. Monitor using an indicator. Slowly rotate at the waist to the right or left until indicator is maximally softened. Maintain until you feel significant softening of indicator.

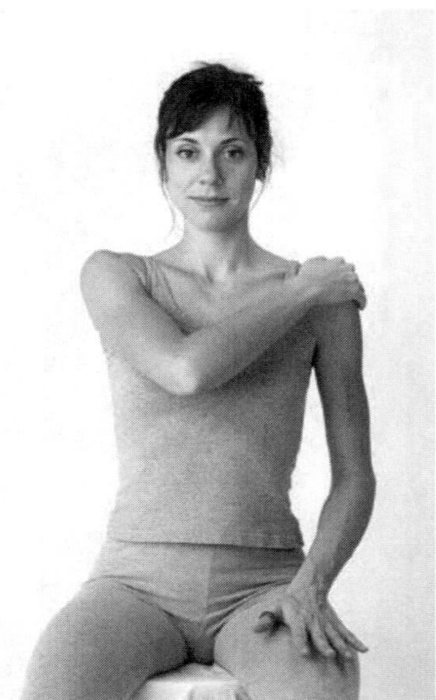

Shoulder: Place hand over primary restriction. Monitor using an indicator. Slowly move the shoulder joint in different directions until indicator is maximally softened. Maintain until you feel significant softening of indicator.

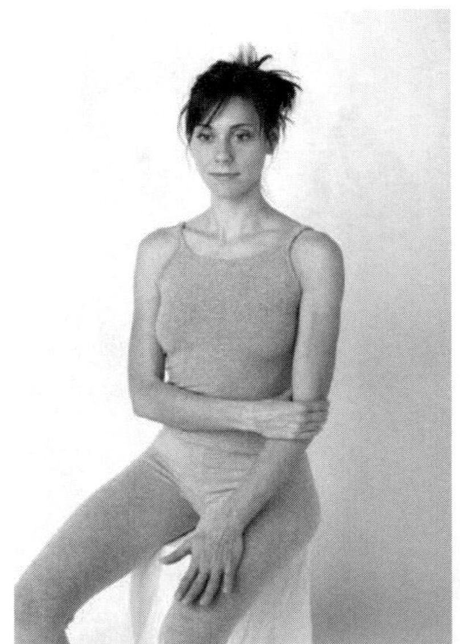

Upper arm: Grasp the end of the upper arm just above the elbow. Monitor using an indicator. Move the bone in different directions until indicator is maximally softened. Maintain until you feel a significant softening of the indicator.

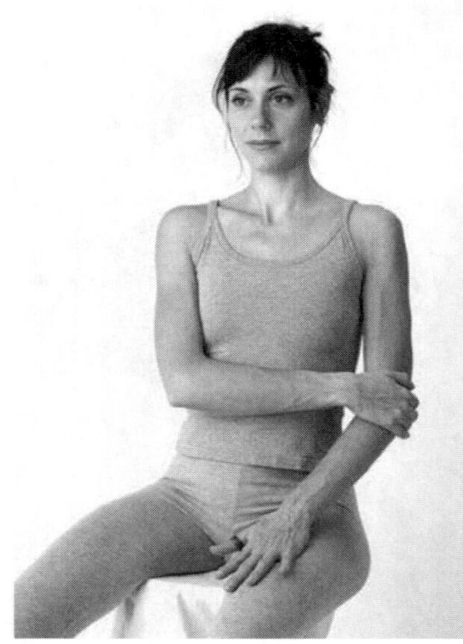

Elbow: Place hand over primary restriction. Monitor using an indicator. Slowly move the elbow joint in different directions, or move it passively by grasping the forearm, until indicator is maximally softened. Maintain until you feel significant softening of indicator.

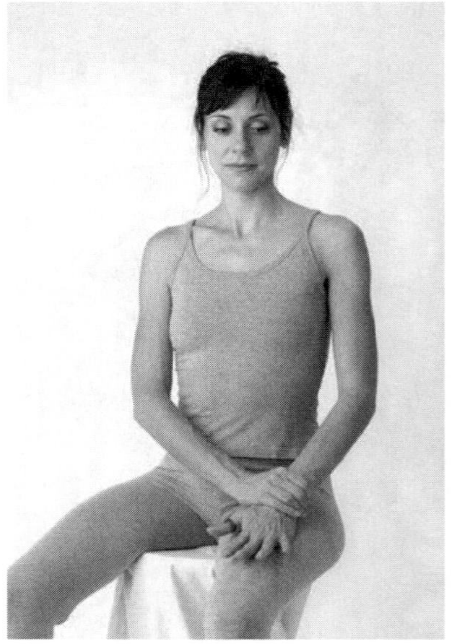

Forearm: Grasp the end of the forearm just above the wrist. Monitor using an indicator. Move the bone in different directions until indicator is maximally softened. Maintain until you feel a significant softening of the indicator.

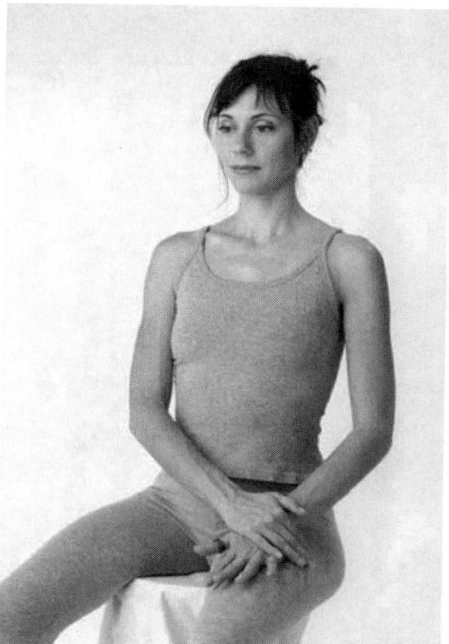

Wrist: Place hand over primary restriction. Monitor using an indicator. Slowly move the wrist joint in different directions, or move it passively by grasping the hand, until indicator is maximally softened. Maintain until you feel significant softening of indicator.

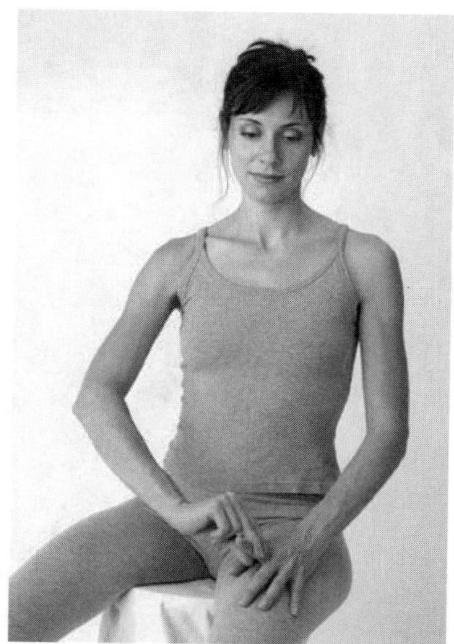

Fingers: Place hand over primary restriction. Monitor using an indicator. Slowly move the finger joint in different directions, or move it passively by grasping the part of the finger farthest from the center of the body, until indicator is maximally softened. Maintain until you feel significant softening of indicator.

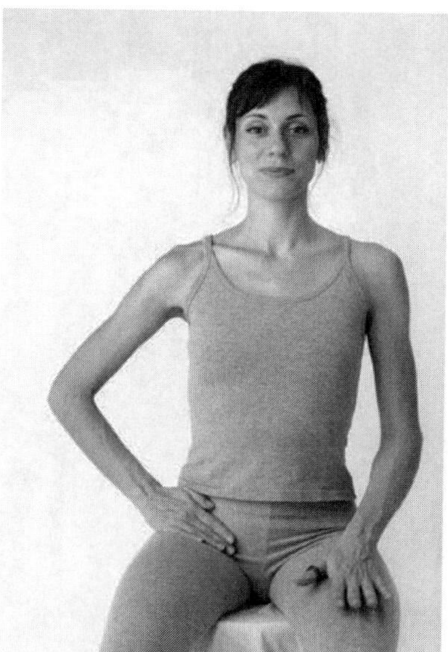

Hip: Place hand over primary restriction. Monitor using an indicator. Slowly move the hip joint in different directions until indicator is maximally softened. Maintain until you feel significant softening of indicator.

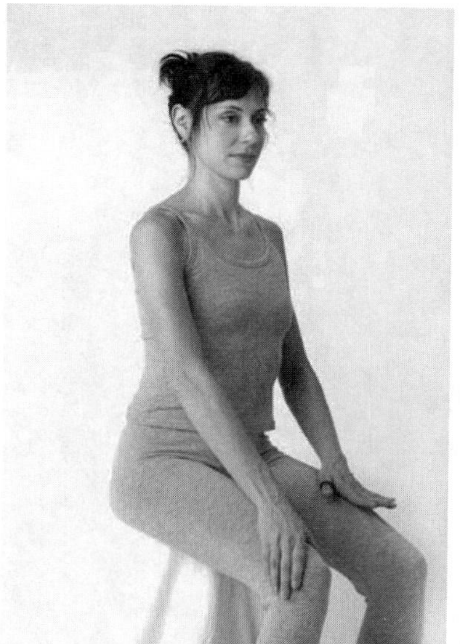

Thigh: Grasp the end of the thigh just above the knee. Monitor using an indicator. Move the bone in different directions until indicator is maximally softened. Maintain until you feel a significant softening of the indicator.

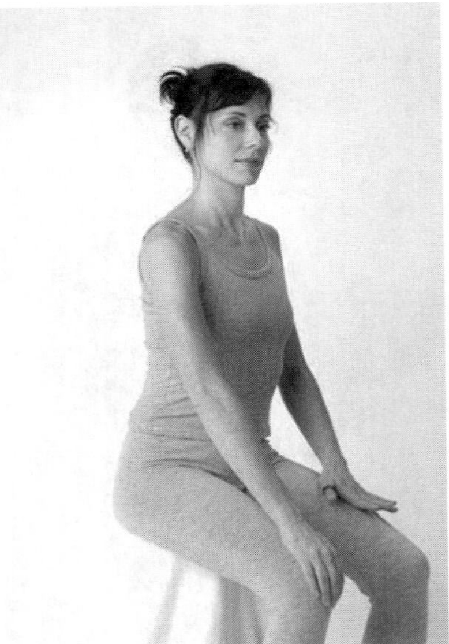

Knee: Place hand over primary restriction. Monitor using an indicator. Slowly move the knee joint in different directions, or move it passively by grasping the leg, until indicator is maximally softened. Maintain until you feel significant softening of indicator.

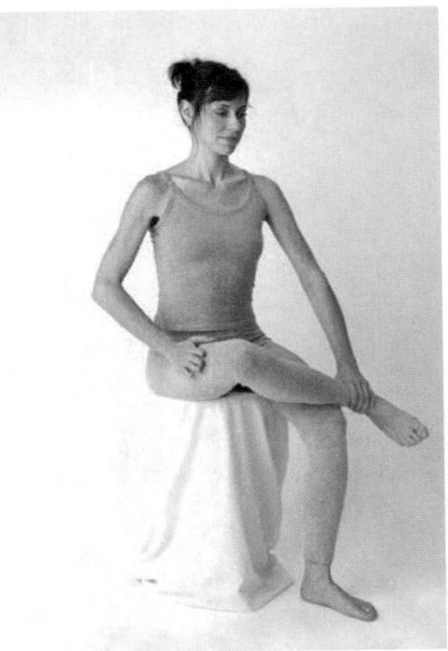

Leg: Grasp the end of the leg just above the ankle. Monitor using an indicator. Move the bone in different directions until indicator is maximally softened. Maintain until you feel a significant softening of the indicator.

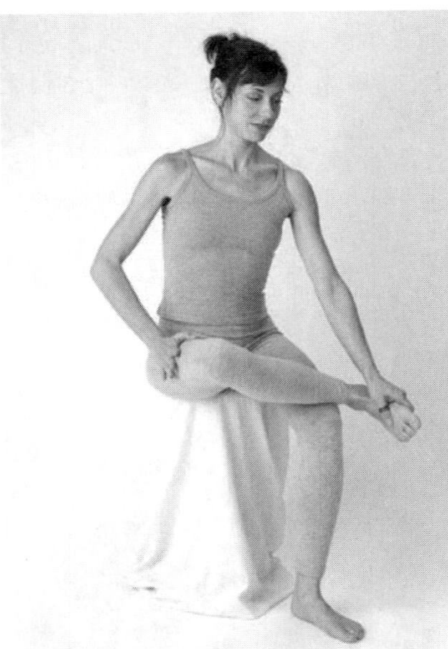

Ankle: Place hand over primary restriction. Monitor using an indicator. Slowly move the ankle joint in different directions, or move it passively by grasping the foot, until indicator is maximally softened. Maintain until you feel significant softening of indicator.

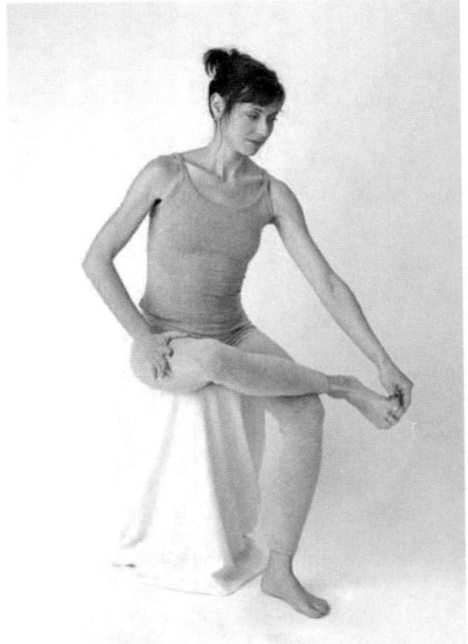

Foot: Place hand over primary restriction. Monitor using an indicator. Slowly move the foot joint in different directions, or move it passively by grasping the part or the foot farthest from the center of the body, until indicator is maximally softened. Maintain until you feel significant softening of indicator.

The Matrix Repatterning Program: Summary

1. **Body Check:** Determine which areas of your body are not moving easily or are out of balance.
2. **Body Scan:** Use the indicator and scan each area listed to determine the priorities among the primary restrictions.
3. **Self-Treatment**:

Electrical Treatment: Place one hand on the primary restriction while monitoring the tension in the indicator. Maintain the contact until a release is felt (significant softening of the indicator or the primary restriction itself.)

Mechanical Treatment: Use the indicator to determine the direction of treatment for bones or joints. Gently hold the position or direction of tension in the area involved until a release is felt.

4. Recheck the areas you found in the Body Check to determine if you have improved the imbalances. Repeat treatment or treat other primary restrictions as indicated.
5. If your pain or limitation persists or worsens, even after following the procedures outlined above, it is recommended that you seek professional assistance.

TREATING KIDS

It's just a fact of life. Every parent knows the routine: Johnny will fall off his bicycle; Mary will slip while skating and hurt her bottom as well as her pride. As a parent, you'll need to tend to bumped knees, bottoms, elbows, and heads and twisted ankles, wrists, and fingers. The daily life of a child can be quite challenging for the child and the parent. How often have you wished you could take away the hurt and offer some real help to your injured child? Ice packs and bandages help, of course, but how about something that could help your child erase the effects of many injuries, so that their active life could resume with out the worry that they might aggravate their condition?

Most of us have been conditioned to connect injury and pain to the fearful prospect of ongoing limitation and declining health. When we stop and realize the real effect of this skewed image of life and how we may have been caught up in this negative perspective, it is easy to understand how our children also might easily pick up on these messages.

Matrix Repatterning principles and techniques, as you apply them to your children, can provide a different message. By restoring the balanced molecular state to the injured area, you support the healing process and the body is less likely to be vulnerable to any lingering effects or reinjury. As your children experience the very real changes you (or they) can create with these simple procedures, they will realize that their bodies are resilient and dependable, that well-being and health are easily restored. This can go a long way to reducing much of the fear associated with injury in the first place.

In order to apply Matrix Repatterning to a child or other family member, start by having them sit or lie down comfortably. Find a suitable indicator. This could be gentle pressure, pushing down on top of their shoulder or on their thigh muscle while they are seated, or pushing gently in on their rib cage while they are lying down. Scan their body according to the list in chapter 4, and note which areas cause a softening of the indicator. Check each primary restriction with the indicator and determine which area causes the most softening. This will be your first treatment priority.

Either maintain the contact over the primary restriction, or have your child do so, for a period of one to five minutes, or until a release is felt. You may be surprised at how sensitive your child is to the changes being made in their body. They may notice how good it feels to have your hand over the area being treated, and when the release occurs, you may notice their breathing deepen, and they may even doze off. They may comment on the effects they are experiencing. It's useful to reinforce the normalcy of all of these responses so they can learn to trust their bodies and their own natural healing abilities.

With certain injuries, the direction of strain or impact is fairly obvious, such as when they fall and land on a knee or elbow, jam a finger, or twist an ankle. Using a mechanical treatment to reverse the direction of injury may then be applied in order to enhance the effectiveness of your treatment.

Over time, you may notice your child automatically treating themselves for various strains and sprains. It is remarkable how quickly they *get* things! Matrix Repatterning is a commonsense approach that often makes sense to kids, especially after they experience the benefits once or twice. And when they notice you have injured yourself or are in any sort of pain, you may be surprised that they then offer to treat you. Relax and enjoy the moment.

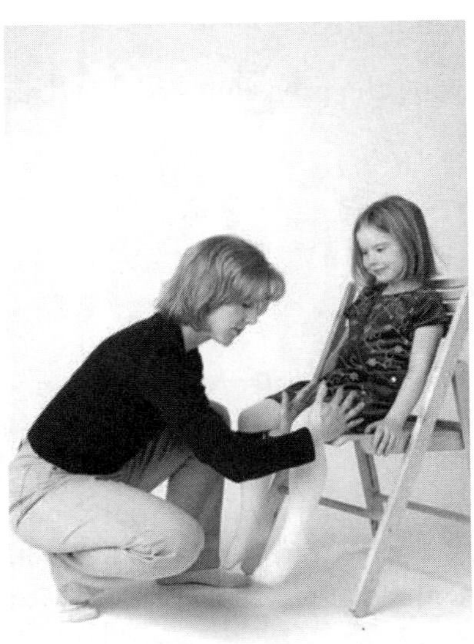

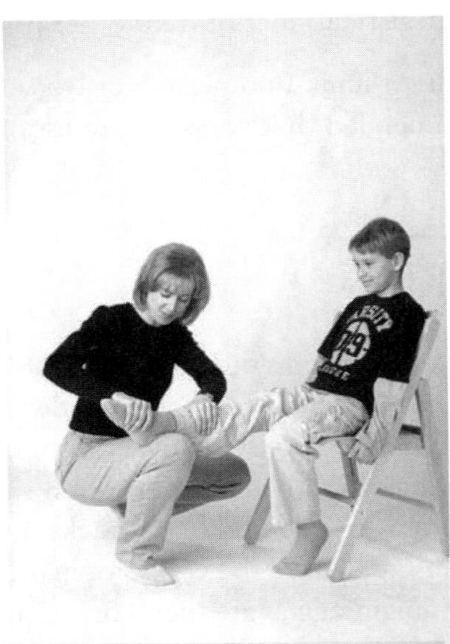

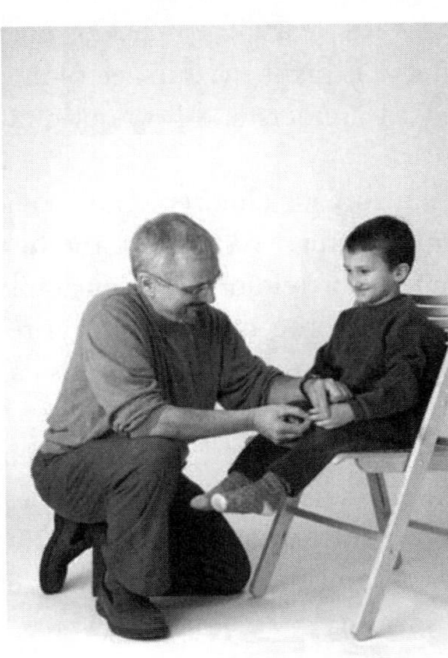

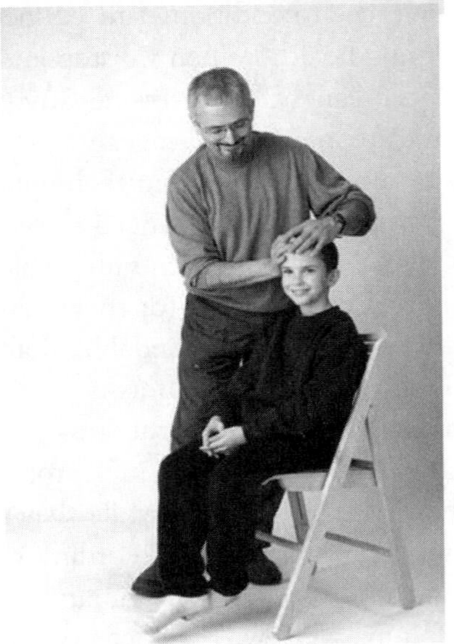

MATRIX REPATTERNING AT WORK AND AT HOME

Our lives are full: housework, career, kids, sports, and other leisure activities. Your body is the vehicle through which you interact with this playground called life. As we now understand, the body is a mechanical apparatus composed of a remarkable, interconnected framework. It is capable of propelling you at great speed, able to lift a surprising amount of weight and move objects in your environment, and help you dance the dance of life with ease and grace. With all this activity, it's not surprising that it is subject to occasional strains or bumps, most of which are easily tolerated without any lingering effects.

On the rare occasion that we encounter a more significant injury, we can use the language of the body to easily determine the source of the imbalance. We can then apply the gentle forms of treatment described in this book to encourage the internal structure of our cells back to their balanced state of structure, thus restoring their ideal state of resilience and function.

Most of us don't have the time to seek professional help every time we encounter one of life's little mishaps. We barely have the time to even pay attention to the aches and pains that often come and go, depending on how much we put our bodies through. It is usually not until a problem becomes annoying enough that we can no longer avoid dealing with it that we may be motivated to find a solution.

The idea of assessing the structure of your own body, searching for primary restrictions, and patiently holding a treatment position may seem a daunting prospect. In most cases, it's not necessary to perform a comprehensive Body Check or even a thorough Body Scan. You can simply check the areas that have been directly affected by an obvious injury. This is also where the Quick Reference Guide for Specific Conditions (chapter 7) may come in handy. By quickly scanning each of the areas listed for a specific problem, which can usually be accomplished in a few minutes, the primary restriction can easily be determined and your treatment can begin.

Many of the treatments can easily be performed while engaged in your normal activities during the day. It is possible, in most cases, to apply the treatment while sitting at your desk or while watching your favorite television program. Taking the time to apply this loving attention to yourself is also a way of relaxing and releasing some of the accumulated mental stress that may build up during your busy day. Sometimes, just setting aside five to ten minutes can restore vitality and renew perspective and clarity. Whether you just sit quietly in a comfortable chair or lie down for a power nap, these time-outs can be of tremendous benefit to your well-being. You can also use these times to apply a Matrix Repatterning Self-Treatment, helping to restore the structure of your body to optimal function at the same time.

The following photos illustrate a few of the comfortable positions that can allow you to provide yourself with a Matrix Repatterning treatment.

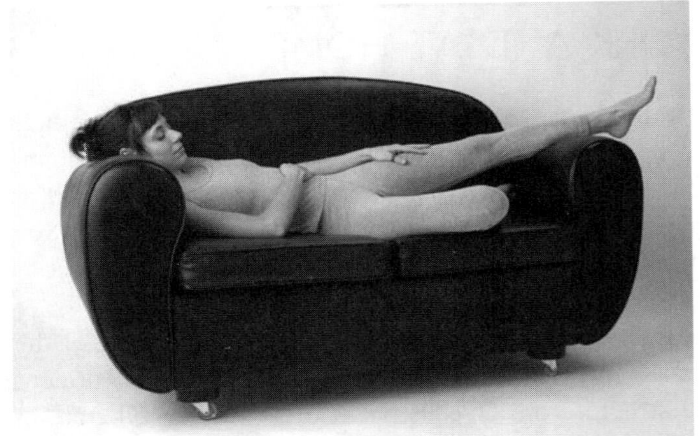

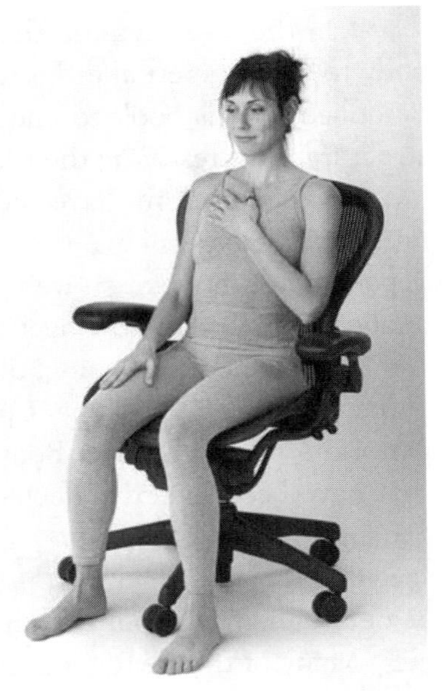

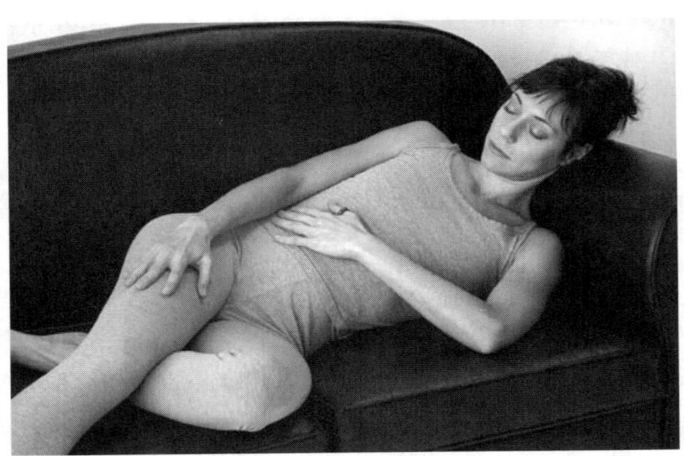

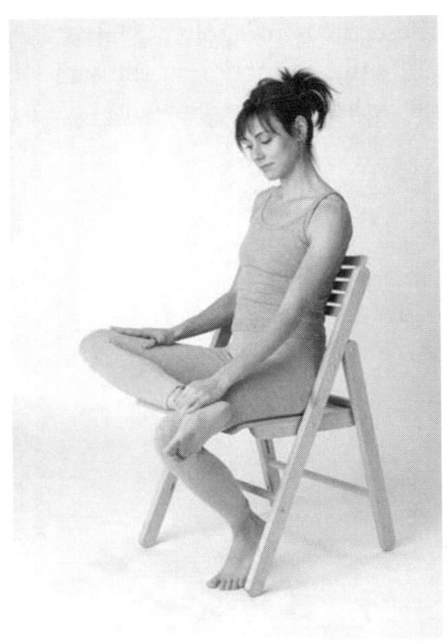

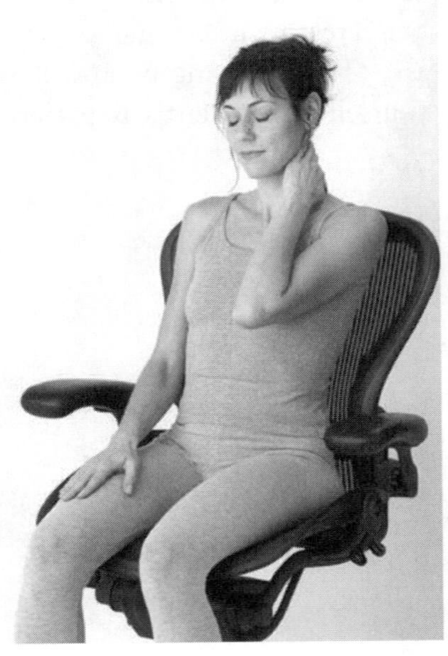

CHAPTER 6

Pain Free at Last

You may have heard about a friend or loved one who has been injured. You may have witnessed their struggle. Sometimes they are able to move forward in their lives, but often they meet with increasing physical limitation and pain. Careers cut short, endless rounds of treatment and medications, health benefits terminated, marriages under increasing financial stress. You may have experienced this in your own life and felt the sense of helplessness and fear that things can only get worse.

A NEW PERSPECTIVE ON HEALTH AND DISEASE

The purpose of this chapter is to help provide you gain a new perspective on the health conditions you may be currently facing or may be worried about. The tensegrity matrix is the way the body is put together, and it defines how the body works. It seems very clear that it is also an important factor in the development of certain diseases. Matrix Repatterning addresses this underlying structure of the body head-on. It can help you to determine the current structural state of your body and help you easily and efficiently restore the balance so vital to optimal health. Of course, this can play an important role in relieving many painful conditions, but it can go much further. Evidence now suggests that the mechanical state of the cells of the body is crucial to general health. Some of this research is even pointing to a role in the major threats to health, including heart disease and cancer (Ingber 1998).

The body has a tremendous capacity to heal itself. When the cells of the body have access to their full potential, they are capable of resisting many illnesses and recovering from illness once it develops. We are not passive receptacles of disease. We have the ability to rally significant resources to help us live long, healthy, and productive lives. Matrix Repatterning can be an important ally in restoring your optimal capacity for self-healing and the maintenance of well-being. Cells are the basis of every tissue in the body, and since cells (and the molecules in them) are being normalized through this process, every part of the body can benefit when they are restored to their ideal state of function. Clear, scientific evidence now suggests that abnormal tension on body tissues, which often results from injury, causes cells to behave abnormally (Ingber 1998). By restoring normal balance and tone to the structure of the body, Matrix Repatterning may also be helpful in maintaining optimal health at the cellular level.

The purpose of Matrix Repatterning is to normalize and support the capacity of every part of the body to function at its optimal level. It is my experience that when the body tissues are restored to their ideal level of tone and balance, they are able to withstand tremendous forces and even resist the tendency to become seriously injured in the first place. It is not the purpose of Matrix Repatterning to heal any condition or to simply alleviate symptoms. The one and only goal of Matrix Repatterning, whether in self-treatment or by a professional, is to precisely locate the sources of the problem (the primary restrictions) and to efficiently and thoroughly release them. The result of doing this will tend to restore normal cell function, which will ultimately allow the body to heal itself. This renders pain—the body's way of alerting us to the fact that something is wrong—unnecessary.

Chronic back pain, arthritis, fibromyalgia, neck pain, headaches, foot problems, knee pain, shoulder pain, carpal tunnel syndrome, and other musculoskeletal conditions usually respond quickly to treatment. Certain cases of digestive complaints, circulatory problems, menstrual pain, abnormal sleep patterns, and other nervous system disturbances, when associated with structural imbalance, may also benefit from Matrix Repatterning. Many people report improved function and increased vitality following treatment. Once the source of the tension is alleviated, the resulting strain in the painful area will significantly improve. The body can then proceed through an accelerated healing process, free of the continuous or repetitive strain imposed by the primary restrictions.

The human frame is unique in the animal world, primarily due to our upright, standing posture. In addition, we have also introduced an array of technological innovations that tend to put us in harm's way: the automobile, high-speed and contact sports, and heavy equipment in industrial settings, to name a few. We are also prone to certain illnesses due to lifestyle choices such as poor diet and sedentary activities. Exposure to chemical toxins and various forms of radiation may impact the cells of your body as well. We may also tend to respond negatively to the demands and stresses of daily life in this highly technological era. Surgical scarring and even the dentist's drill can become important factors in the development of primary restrictions.

The human condition can be challenging at times. Illness and pain can make us especially vulnerable to losing our perspective, making it difficult to see beyond the immediate limitations we are facing. Stories about others who have shared similar challenges and who have been able to overcome their conditions can give us hope and inspire us to persevere in our quest to rise above our pain and fear. The stories in this chapter are about people like you who have experienced pain and disability and who have found their way back, through Matrix Repatterning, to a life of freedom and vitality. It is my hope that these accounts will serve to inspire you to find your way back to the life that you intended to live, in all its fullness and joy.

SPINAL CONDITIONS: A REAL PAIN IN THE NECK (AND BACK)

Back and neck pain—most people have had it at some time in their life. When you have it, it seems like you're going to be crippled for the rest of your life. In most cases, after resting for one to three weeks, the pain subsides and life resumes. After that, you gradually get back into your normal routine with no pain. Eventually you forget that horrible experience—until the next time! Then *bam*—it hits you again. You have now entered the ranks of the back pain sufferers, and the fear of future attacks looms over you like a snake in the branches, ready to pounce on you without warning.

Scientists have sliced, imaged, dissected, computerized, and pulverized pieces of the spine, trying to uncover the cause of back and neck pain.

You start reading about other sufferers and the myriad theories and tactics to avoid and/or treat this condition. Your life begins to become limited by the fear of another round of debilitating pain and so you don't pick up your kids anymore, you choose the less challenging ski slopes (if at all), and you baby yourself with every little twinge. In general, you begin to distrust your body and wonder if this is the beginning of the slippery slope.

The next stage, after experiencing several episodes of back pain, is the search for solutions at any cost. You trudge along to various specialists of every description. You get stretched, cracked, prodded, poked, scalded and, yes, you even feel some delicious relief, for a while. Then the pain returns. You try several different medications and are now even considering that step into the abyss—surgery. The word itself is enough to strike terror into the most courageous of us. You're put to sleep, and a bunch of high-tech equipment is attached to your body while someone cuts into you and rearranges pieces of your anatomy. You may even feel some relief after the shock wears off. But, just as likely, the condition returns, often with some new, added (and unwelcome) twists. You begin to wonder where it will all end.

Endless Theories

The spine has been the subject of an enormous amount of scientific study and debate. It has been estimated that approximately 80 percent of North Americans will experience some significant back or neck pain before the age of forty. Scientists have sliced, imaged, dissected, computerized, and pulverized pieces of the spine, trying to uncover the cause of back and neck pain. Doctors, therapists, and various other clinicians have fused, cut out, injected, bolted, inserted rods, pummeled, cracked, stretched, twisted, and exercised ad infinitum in the elusive attempt to alleviate this age-old affliction.

The advent of the X-ray presented the spine as a disembodied stack of bones, separated by disks and other soft tissues invisible to the X-ray. The apparent misalignment of the vertebrae and/or the collapse of the spaces between them led to the conclusion that this "fragile" and frequently imbalanced structure must be the source of the patient's condition.

The spine is richly supplied with position, movement, and pain nerve receptors of every description. Stimulation of some of the pain nerve endings can even reproduce the patient's complaints. Some theories have been put forward that these nerve endings must, in some way, be directly responsible for the condition. Several therapies have been designed to relieve pressure on nerves or to inject them with pain-numbing drugs. One "innovative" method even offers to relieve the pain by surgically removing the offending pain nerve fibers themselves! Killing the messenger?

The bottom line: There is an abysmal track record for all of these theories and therapies. In most cases, any relief attained is short-lived. Worse yet, the deterioration of the spine continues and general functioning and the ability to resume normal activities of life and work are not improved.

A New Perspective

The integrity of the spinal cord (the bundle of nerves connecting the brain to every other part of the body) is essential to every aspect of the coordinated functioning of the body. Without it, we would be unable to move, feed ourselves, or even maintain the functioning of many of our organs. The bones of the spine (the vertebrae) protect the delicate spinal cord housed within it. The numerous joints of the spine are designed to give in response to strain. They possess complex movement capabilities, which provide an essential role in diverting any structural imbalances from potentially damaging the vulnerable tissues of the spinal cord. The spine is, in fact, very well designed to reduce the potentially damaging forces that could threaten the individual's life.

Let us consider the spine from the perspective of the tensegrity structural model and Matrix Repatterning. As part of the interconnected fascial (fibrous) matrix of the body, the spine, like any other part of the body, would be subject to any and all abnormal strain patterns arising from any one of a number of possible primary restrictions anywhere in the body. The painful signals being relayed to the brain from the spine may be an attempt to warn that a particular range of motion could potentially damage the spinal cord or the spinal nerves. This could jeopardize the individual's ability to feed, escape predators, and even reproduce.

The distorted positions of the vertebrae, seen on an X-ray, are often simply an expression of this protective response (Levin 2002; Masi and Walsh 2003). In many cases, the actual source of the spinal imbalance is arising from somewhere other than the spine itself. The primary source of tension therefore pulls on the tensegrity matrix, which in turn pulls on the spine. This leads to abnormal patterns of movement of the spinal joints, causing local pain, and may also lead to the wear and tear and resulting deterioration of the spinal disk (cushions between the vertebrae) and the joints.

Another spinal component (often overlooked by most practitioners) is the membrane surrounding the spinal cord, referred to as the *meninges*. This fluid-filled structure is particularly vulnerable to impact and straining forces common in many types of injuries. Meningeal strain may be the source of spinal pain and other structural or neurological conditions. Specific Matrix Repatterning techniques are designed to address restrictions within this structure.

From the perspective of the interconnected tensegrity matrix, the pain in the spine itself may have nothing to do with the source of the problem. The spine may simply be reacting to the overall structural imbalance being expressed throughout the body and performing its overriding function of protecting the delicate nerve pathways housed within it. Fortunately the treatment strategies of Matrix Repatterning can address the true source of the problem, no matter where in the body it lies. Read the following two stories to see how this can work.

Jill's Story: Overcoming Low-Back Pain

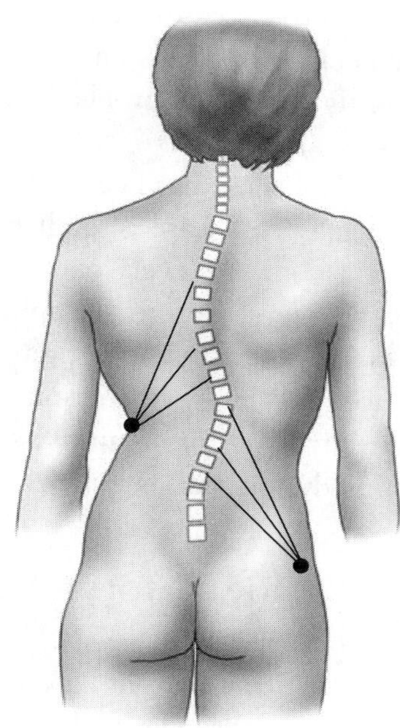

Figure 6-1: Spinal strain patterns

Jill was thirty-one years old. She developed acute low back pain that included pain radiating into the front of her left thigh and into her right leg and the top of her right foot. These pains were made worse by sitting, bending forward, and bending sideways to the right. She had to use her arms to support the weight of her body while sitting in order to avoid pressure. She had experienced two previous episodes dating back seven years since a severe fall on her tailbone after slipping on the deck of a boat. Since that injury, she'd had low back stiffness and moderate pain between these acute episodes. She had been receiving regular chiropractic care over the years.

My examination revealed extremely limited forward bending and side bending to the right. The joints between the base of her spine and her hips (sacroiliac joints) were stuck and her tailbone (coccyx) was deformed due to the force of the impact of her original injury. Her low back and knee joints were moving excessively, as I often find when the bones of the pelvis are injured. Her liver and right kidney were stuck in an expanded state, and her right kidney was positioned lower than normal. Nerve tests were normal.

I applied treatment to the sacroiliac, sacrum, kidney, and liver. When I re-examined her, she had a 50 percent improvement in the movement of her low back, the joints of her low back and left knee were stabilized, and she was able to sit comfortably for the first time in over a week. Follow-up therapy was directed at scar tissue resulting from two previous abdominal surgeries. After four treatments, Jill was completely symptom free, and her ranges of motion were normal.

Harold's Story: Neck Pain, No Problem

Harold was forty-eight years old. He came to my office with a complaint of neck pain of over ten year's duration. He had a history of numerous sports injuries from hockey and skiing falls. He had received extensive and repeated chiropractic care over the years, as well as physical therapy—all to no avail.

My examination revealed very tight neck muscles, especially on the left. The joints in the middle of his neck were pulled out of position and were very tender to the touch. His ability to turn his neck to the left and bend it to the right were reduced. I found four primary restrictions: the left thighbone was compressed (a common sequel to a fall on the knee), the left hip bone was compressed and widened (the result of the common injury of falling sideways onto the hip), the left kidney was expanded (remember, the dense, water-filled organs are common victims of impact injuries and are often a missed part of the diagnosis of musculoskeletal problems), and the fourth area of involvement was in the shoulder due to a previous fall onto his side.

I directed treatment to the primary restrictions over two sessions. The apparent neck strain was completely resolved on re-examination. Range of motion was restored, and the rigid muscle tension was normalized. Harold has had no further complaints of neck pain in over two years since treatment was rendered.

Harold's case is typical of the types of undiagnosed primary restrictions that can easily alter spinal biomechanics. The spine is a potential source of dysfunction, but I have found that it is much less frequently the actual problem than would be assumed from the amount of therapy traditionally directed to this area.

The spine has been a central theme in many medical specialties. The fact that it is often the site of pain may be a case of guilt by association. If we consider the true nature of the tensegrity matrix and how it connects every part of the body to every other part, we must consider many other possibilities as the source of pain in the spine. It has been my experience and that of many of my students, that when therapy is directed appropriately to the source of the dysfunction, spinal biomechanics are often instantly restored. Primary restrictions of the spine do exist, but based on the new information about the underlying structure of organic tissue, we should keep an open mind and consider that the primary source of spinal dysfunction may lie elsewhere.

■ Joe's Story: Low Back Pain Solved—and a Surprise

Joe arrived for his appointment and described the low back pain that had been plaguing him for over six months. His work as a tool-and-die maker required lots of twisting and bending. He found he was eventually unable to work without excruciating pain. Typical of many men, he waited until he was practically crawling on his hands and knees before, at the insistence of his wife, he sought out help.

When I examined him, I found some of the typical issues that might be related to his condition: pelvic imbalance, a knee-injury pattern, and significant primary restrictions in both of his kidneys and his liver. Primary restrictions in the organs are very common from falls and other impact injuries, which had certainly been part of his history from his years of playing amateur hockey. I proceeded to treat him on the first visit for several of these issues and had him schedule a follow-up appointment in a week's time.

When Joe arrived the following week, he mentioned how much better his back felt, and then he asked me an interesting question:

"I was wondering if your treatment might have caused something else?"

"What do you mean?" I asked rather apprehensively.

"Well, I've had heartburn for about nine years. I've tried many types of drugs, but nothing has really helped me."

"I see. And what does that have to do with the treatment we did last week?" I invited him to continue his story.

"Well, that's just it. I mean my back is almost perfect since then, but my heartburn—I think the doctor called it reflux . . ."

"Yes, gastroesophageal reflux or GERD" I offered.

"Yeah, that's it. That's what he called it."

"So, what happened to your reflux?" I asked.

"Well, it's gone!" He threw up his hands, and his eyes lit up. "Could that be because of the treatment? I mean, I have not had a whole week without this problem in over nine years. Is it possible?"

I smiled back at his obvious delight in his new-found freedom from this often debilitating condition. "Yes, it certainly is possible, and it's not the first time I have heard of someone with that kind of experience. You see, when you have a structural imbalance and it's affecting certain internal organs around the diaphragm—that's the umbrella-shaped muscle above your stomach—correcting these organs often normalizes the tension around the opening of the swallowing tube—the esophagus—to the stomach. If this opening is not working properly, it may allow acid from the stomach to splash up into the esophagus, which is not designed to handle these acids. That's why it causes you to experience the burning sensation."

He nodded in understanding.

"So, if you balance the tensions in these areas of the body," I continued "then the opening can also work the way it was designed."

"Wow, it's just great!" Joe continued. "I have even been able to eat some of my favorite sausage this week. I just couldn't believe it."

"I'm glad to hear that Joe. You might want to go easy for a while, until your stomach has had a chance to get used to things." I suggested.

"No problem, doc. Thanks!" Joe said as he got up to leave. "I'll let you know how things go."

I heard from Joe a few months later when he called to make an appointment for his son. He said his back—and his stomach—were still just fine.

Scoliosis

Scoliosis is an abnormal, side-to side curvature of the spine. On an X-ray, the spine of a person with scoliosis looks more like an "S" or a "C" than a straight line. Some of the bones in a spine with scoliosis also may have rotated slightly, making the person's waist or shoulders appear uneven. It appears to develop mysteriously, mainly in adolescent females. Many people have no pain associated with it, while in more severe cases it may result in progressive deformity, as well as pain and organ problems throughout life.

I have encountered a number of people with this condition and have valiantly sought to ease their pain. Before I discovered Matrix Repatterning, I was never so bold as to assume that I could alter the essential pattern of accentuated curvatures and vertebral deformation reminiscent of this spinal condition. However I tried to release some of the tension in the spinal muscles associated with it. It seemed, however, that all my efforts were casually resisted by this tenacious condition.

■ Liz's Story: Correcting Scoliosis by Accident

When I first encountered a patient with significant scoliosis, since having discovered some of these basic principles, I had no intention of performing any miracles. Liz was a thirty-two-year-old mother of three children. She had complaints of low back, hip, and neck pain. She also had a previously diagnosed scoliosis resulting in the typical S-shaped deformity.

On the first visit I performed my usual assessment and proceeded to treat her for the primary restrictions, which I found in the right kidney, the liver, the left side of the her pelvis, and her left thigh bone. When I retested Liz, her range of motion improved immediately, and she reported less pain with motion. I then asked her to lie down on the table so that I could recheck her for any further areas that might be involved. As she lay down on the table, she exclaimed, "What did you do to me?" Well, you can imagine what went through my mind. I hadn't done anything traumatic, but I wondered if I had done anything to hurt her.

Feigning calm confidence, I reluctantly inquired as to the nature of her exclamation. She responded, "I have never been able to lie flat on a table before. What did you do?" I asked her if she had any pain. She reported that she did not. I proceeded to have her stand up, and much to my amazement, her previously obvious spinal deformity was now almost nonexistent.

I was both shocked and delighted. I had encountered some remarkable results using Matrix Repatterning, however, I had not seen such an extreme case of spinal deformity—apparently structural in nature—disappear, literally before my eyes. I followed her case for some time after this, along with some minor fine-tuning treatment. To date, five years later, she has not had any noticeable return of her scoliosis.

I have seen a number of people over the years with varying degrees of this condition, and so far, have not been able to make any general conclusions on any one set of causes. I have had good results with several cases and mixed results with others.

Scoliosis may be the result of falls and other impact injury incurred during adolescence. The individuals I have encountered admitted to being tomboys in that phase of their lives. These largely undetected effects of injury could, in theory, lead to this type of spinal deformity. Based on some limited experience with this condition, I believe that there is some real hope that this and many other structural conditions may be resolvable. Recent evidence suggests that certain patterns of tension may be attributable to emotional issues during puberty. I am still pursuing further study in this area.

THE PELVIS—GETTING TO THE BOTTOM OF THE PROBLEM

Our high center of gravity makes us vulnerable to forces that tend to destabilize us from the vertical posture. In other words, we tend to fall on our rears with great regularity. This somewhat painful and embarrassing event is usually brushed aside, and as the initial discomfort subsides, we tend to ignore any persisting symptoms until they, too, diminish. However, when we look closely at the dynamics of this type of injury, we can see the potentially large forces involved and the seriousness of the possible long-term effects.

The pelvis consists of three large bones (right and left pelvic bones and the bottom of the spine, called the *sacrum*), all of the surrounding muscles, ligaments, and tendons, the internal organs housed within it, and the fibrous tissue holding everything together. When you fall onto part of this structure, you actually impact onto a small corner of the outer pelvis, usually only two to three square inches of bone, depending on how you land. This impact converts the weight of a one-hundred-and-fifty-pound adult into hundreds of pounds of force per square inch, creating a tremendous impact on the pelvic structures. This type of injury is extremely common and may be the primary cause of mechanical imbalances leading to many cases of low back, hip, and knee problems. Since the internal organs of the pelvis may be directly affected by the abnormal tension due to these injuries, certain conditions affecting the reproductive system, the urinary tract (including the prostate), erectile dysfunction, and the lower intestine, may also be associated with these patterns. Consider Samuel's experience.

■ Samuel's Story: Olympic Dreams

Samuel was discovered on the rugby field by a track-and-field coach. The coach was amazed at the young man's speed and agility, and he approached the young man and asked him to try out for the team. When Samuel was clocked in the one-hundred-meter sprint, the coach couldn't believe his eyes.

This untrained young athlete could have ranked in the top ten in the world without so much as one hour's formal training.

Samuel decided to join the track team and was immediately put into training for the next Olympics. Within a few months, however, disaster struck. Samuel was felled by an excruciating groin injury that, despite months of intensive therapy, would not respond to treatment.

His trainer had just recently taken one of my seminars and decided to refer him to me for assessment. I have always found athletes to be an inspiration to discover new and better ways of treating the body. Samuel's case was no exception. I found several features of injuries he had probably sustained in previous years on the rugby field. Rugby is a notably rough sport, and serious injuries are common. In Samuel's case, a number of impacts to the bones of the pelvis and knees had taken their toll. These impacts had resulted in molecular changes in the bones of the pelvis. Also, since the pelvis contains a significant amount of fluid (all of the organs of the lower abdomen), many of these injuries had resulted in explosive fluid expansion, which had distorted his pelvic structure from the inside. These combined effects had resulted in his persistent symptoms.

Within four sessions to correct each of these injury patterns, Samuel was able to return to training after more than six months of disability. He is now well on his way to competing at the summer Olympics and a brilliant career in track and field.

LOWER LIMBS

■ Cheryl's Story: Healing a Lower Limb

Cheryl was a forty-six-year-old kindergarten teacher and the ultimate skeptic. She was in my office under duress, because her friend was unrelenting in encouraging her to come. She had suffered with knee pain for over twenty years after falling onto some rocks when she was twenty-five. Her left knee appeared swollen. She told me that it became enlarged after the accident and that it caused her continual pain ever since that day.

I examined her carefully and acknowledged that her knee was somewhat swollen but saw that most of the enlargement was because the end of her thighbone (her femur) had changed it's shape. I told her that Matrix Repatterning could probably improve that and help her knee to function more normally. She was new to my ideas and wasn't impressed with my explanation of the tensegrity matrix or my assertion that I could change the shape and function of her knee.

I explained that the treatment would not be painful and there was no risk involved. She shrugged her shoulders to convey her less-than-enthusiastic acquiescence to being treated. I used some calipers to measure the end of the femur and found that the injured bone was over one inch larger in diameter than the uninjured side. I showed her the measurements. She shrugged.

I proceeded to release the tension in her femur, both the enlarged head and the shortened shaft, as well as several other components of that and other injuries. It was at that point that I noticed that her eyes and mouth had popped open. She was flabbergasted.

"What happened?" Was all she could stammer.

"What do you mean?" I asked.

"My knee—it's different. It's not as big!" she exclaimed.

"Well, let's see." I said nonchalantly. I got out my trusty calipers and remeasured the ends of her knees. "Mmm." I said, "They're both the same size now. How about that!"

"That's amazing." Was all she could manage. "I didn't believe that was possible."

I chuckled to myself at her sudden enthusiasm. I explained that bone was just like all other tissues of the body. When it is compressed or strained, the arrangement of its molecules appears to change its shape. Matrix Repatterning, since it works on the primary source of this molecular reaction, appears to often instantly restore the normal shape to these structures.

Subsequent to that treatment, Cheryl experienced complete relief from her nagging knee problems. She can still barely believe it.

The lower limb (thigh, leg, and foot) in the human, two-legged animal is a complex structure—a compromise between mobility and stability. Gravity is always at work to topple the arrogant human who dares to stand on two feet instead of four. Due to the amount of force created when our upright posture and the force of gravity meet head-on, the lower half of our body often sustains a significant amount of injury. Falling on the long bones of the leg and thigh can easily create a change in the molecular structure within the bone itself (we call this an *intraosseous*—within the bone—*lesion*). It's not uncommon to see a measurable change in the bones of the lower limb after an injury. A person who falls on their knee often experiences an enlargement of one-quarter to over one inch in the diameter of the end of the femur (thighbone). This effect is caused by the spreading out or flattening of the molecules near the end of the bone. The net result of an impact to the end of a long bone is an overall shortening and a "mushrooming" or widening of one or both ends. The joints around these bones are therefore subject to significant mechanical stress and abnormal wear-and-tear (see osteoarthritis below).

The forces generated when we are knocked over or when we fall can be extreme. The foot may be planted on the ground as something or someone comes hurtling at us (contact sports enthusiasts are particularly vulnerable), so the rest of the body above the point of impact is jackknifed. The knees, hips, and low back are often the victims of this kind of injury. A strain (or overstretch) that elongates the bones and joints of the lower limb can occur when the foot catches on an obstruction as the person falls forward while the foot remains fixed. This type of strain can also occur in skiing injuries in which the bindings do not immediately release during a fall. The ski and the foot attached to it remain relatively fixed on the slope, leaving the rest of the unfortunate skier to hurtle forward until brought up sharply by the attachment. The leg, ankle, and foot are also prone to bending or twisting injuries due to missteps or certain sports injuries.

The concept of bone responding to injury force—short of actual fracture—is novel within most branches of the healing arts. But when the practitioner takes the trouble to examine the normal resiliency of the bones and the relative dimensions of one limb versus the other, they often begin to extend their belief system to include this important component as part of their assessment. The frequency of primary restrictions in the bones of the lower and upper limbs may come as a surprise to the uninitiated. The density of bone in relation to other tissues and its tendency to absorb traumatic forces is a simple application of basic physics. Bone is not the rigid material we have all come to believe. It is plastic in nature and an important potential source of disturbed patterns of tension in the body.

UPPER LIMBS

The upper limb (arm, forearm, and hand) has a similar structure to the lower limb. It is subject to a different set of traumatic forces, which often involve the breaking of a fall. The hand, wrist, and forearm are particularly vulnerable to injury in this situation. A similar injury can occur when the person lands on their elbow. These injuries, like those of the lower limb, cause changes in the shape of the bones, usually a shortening of the shaft and a widening (mushrooming) of the ends of the bone. A fall onto the side may involve a blow to the tip of the shoulder. In this case, the head of the upper arm (*humerus*), the collar bone (*clavicle*), and the shoulder blade (*scapula*) take the brunt of the force and will become primary sources of the injury complex. The hands and fingers are also subject to trauma due to falls and direct blows during sports activities and in industrial settings.

As in all cases of pain or disturbed function of one part of the body, the source of the problem—the primary restrictions—may lie elsewhere. Many conditions of the upper limb including joint pain, restricted movement, weakness, numbness or tingling, or so-called carpal tunnel syndrome may be due to primary restrictions within the internal organs of the trunk or elsewhere in the body.

So-called "frozen shoulder" is a condition that has frustrated many practitioners of physical medicine. A study on the use of Matrix Repatterning in six cases of frozen shoulder was presented (Roth 2000). The results demonstrated a significant improvement in range of motion with an average of six treatments. This illustrated, once again, that treating the primary source of the problem in many conditions can lead to positive outcomes.

■ Alex's Story: Self-Treatment for Arm Pain

Alex woke up one morning and reached over to turn off his alarm clock. A sudden jolt of pain went through his shoulder like a lightning bolt. He ignored the insistent alarm while he rubbed his now-throbbing arm.

He spent the next few weeks babying his arm. Opening doors, pulling on his jacket, and even reaching for items on the shelf at work resulted in almost paralyzing jolts of pain that abruptly stopped him in his tracks. He consulted a physical therapist and a chiropractor, but after six weeks of therapy he was no further ahead.

A friend happened to mention the self-treatment seminars at our clinic. He read about Matrix Repatterning on our Web site and decided to give it a try. At the seminar he watched the introductory video and learned how to use the indicator to locate his primary restrictions. He asked the instructor to verify his self-assessment. He found a primary restriction over the center of his chest and proceeded to treat it. When he was done he noticed that his arm felt less tender when he moved it in different directions. However, he still noticed some sharp pain when he reached over his head.

He decided to check himself one more time for any more primary restrictions. He located another one over a tooth on the same side as his sore arm. With the instructor's help, he was able to pinpoint the most significant area. He poked at it and noticed how tender it was. He recalled how that tooth had been sensitive to hot and cold over the past few months. He relaxed into a comfortable position with his hand over the side of his face. His other hand continued to monitor the indicator in his thigh muscle. After a few minutes, he noticed that his thigh muscle relaxed a lot more. It was almost as if it had melted!

He checked the movement in his arm once again and was surprised to see that he was able to move it in all directions with practically no pain at all. When the seminar was over, his Matrix Repatterning instructor reminded the class to keep an open mind about where the primary restrictions might be located. They were also instructed to pay attention to any aggravation of their condition, and that if it did not improve within five to seven days to consult with their health professional.

Alex performed the self-assessment and treatment process two more times over the course of the following week and found that his arm pain was completely gone. He was pleased to notice that his tooth was also no longer sensitive.

This story can serve to remind us of the power each of us has to take charge of our own health. With a very simple procedure, Alex was able to locate and treat several of the primary restrictions that were contributing to his pain. He had discovered his own self-healing capabilities and was able to resolve a condition that was seriously interfering with his life through the use of Matrix Repatterning principles.

ARTHRITIS

Arthritis literally means "inflammation of a joint." It can be caused from any source of irritation, and as such, is a very nonspecific diagnosis. The most common forms of this condition are osteoarthritis and rheumatoid arthritis.

Osteoarthritis

Osteoarthritis is a form of arthritis marked by the degeneration of the cartilage and bone joints. As you have read above, bone is subject to direct injury that can alter its shape and mechanical properties. It is possible that some of the pain and inflammation associated with osteoarthritis may be due to this primary distortion of the bone (Duncan 1995). Most common sites include the knee, spine, hip, ankle, wrist, and hand. Surgery is sometimes recommended for this condition, even though current studies indicate it is often ineffective (Mosley et al. 2002).

This condition may also be caused by the mechanical imbalances imposed on the joints by primary restrictions elsewhere in the body, leading to abnormal joint function and wear and tear on the delicate components of the joint. Matrix Repatterning practitioners have found that addressing these underlying causes of mechanical imbalance can often lead to improved joint function and reduction of inflammation in the affected joints. More long-term studies are needed to verify these factors.

Rheumatoid Arthritis

Rheumatoid arthritis is a systemic (throughout the body) condition representing a general autoimmune condition affecting many tissues, including the joints. Matrix Repatterning may offer some symptom relief in these cases. General treatment addressing primary restrictions throughout the body may also assist the functioning of various organs. This may provide some assistance toward restoring a state of physiologic balance within the body, which may help to alleviate certain aspects of the general state of health contributing to this illness.

MUSCLES, LIGAMENTS, AND TENDONS

The power to interact with the environment—running, jumping, hunting, gathering, tilling the soil, playing the piano, dancing, embracing, and smiling—has the power of movement at its very core. The ability to perform these activities is one of the defining features of human life and something we generally take for granted until it is impaired or taken away.

Muscles are the prime movers of the body. They are made of an amazing complex of proteins and fibrous tissue giving them the capacity to contract with tremendous force. They are connected to the brain by way of nerves that not only initiate the contraction of the muscle fibers but also provide constant feedback about the loads being lifted or the degree to which the body part has moved in space. Muscles attach to bone by way of strong bundles of fibrous tissue called *tendons*. The joints are also part of this impressive array of feedback systems allowing the body to move smoothly, gracefully, and with significant power. The thick fibrous strands that hold joints together and guide their movements are called *ligaments*.

Healthy muscle is supple and has a wide range of tolerance to stretch. Injury, such as a significant strain or a sudden, unexpected increase in loading, can lead to a primary restriction within the muscle, its tendons, or the ligaments within the joint. This often results in a reactive spasm of the muscle itself and an overstretching of the tendons and ligaments. This can result in a loss of flexibility or an alteration of the normal abilities of the muscle to contract, relax, or simply to support that part of the body. The ligaments may lose their ability to maintain stability within the joints, resulting in abnormal movement patterns and subsequent wear and tear of the delicate internal joint structures. These changes are often accompanied by pain, swelling, inflammation, and local tenderness (Lewitt 1985).

Most so-called muscle strain is usually the result of prolonged or moderately elevated stress on a muscle beyond its normal capacity. This may result in the stimulation of some of the stretch and/or pain nerve endings in the coverings (fascia) around the muscle or a build-up of excess waste products within the muscle, leading to stimulation of the chemical pain receptors. In each of these instances, rest is all that is required to restore the tissues to their normal state. Conditioning exercises are valuable in preparing muscles for increased workloads, and within a relatively short period of time, an activity that previously may have resulted in strain or pain may be well tolerated with no ill effects.

Several conditions are associated with pain in the muscles and their fascia. The term *fibromyalgia* is simply a union of three Greek words meaning "pain in the fibrous and muscular tissues" (see the section below on fibromyalgia). Unfortunately, the diagnosis does not indicate the source of the problem, although several unproven theories are in the current literature (Rachlin 1994). Other terms such as *myofascial pain syndrome*, *tension myositis syndrome,* and *fibrositis* have been used. Each of these conditions is typified by pain and inflammation in the muscles, tendons, and ligaments—the so-called soft tissue elements of the musculoskeletal system.

From the Matrix Repatterning point of view, many of these cases are simply the direct result of abnormal tension transmitted through the matrix, resulting in strain and irritation in one or more areas. Muscles working against constant or repetitive resistance and ligaments trying to control joints that are moving in ways for which they were not designed will naturally become irritated and set up a chronic state of inflammation.

In addition to the abnormal mechanical forces exerted by primary restrictions within the matrix, Ingber and others have pointed out the very real physiological changes at the cellular level initiated by abnormal tension on the molecular structure. The cell, now distorted by mechanical tension, begins to behave in ways that may also cause it to alter its biochemical function, including the release of chemical mediators of inflammation. The cells and the tissues in which they exist may become disturbed in their function (Ingber 1998). Matrix Repatterning practitioners have found that restoring the normal mechanical state to the tissues often results in the normalization of muscle and joint function.

SPORTS INJURIES

From the weekend warrior to the elite athlete, humankind is constantly striving for the sheer pleasure of expressing the joy of living through physical activity. Pushing, pulling, jumping, running, lifting, spinning, sliding, bouncing—and yes, falling, crashing, smashing, and slashing—are all a part of life on the edge. We wouldn't want it any other way.

Every sport has a unique set of variables and risks, just as every athlete is unique in their abilities and susceptibility to injury. Joint strains and impact injuries are the most common complaints. Dealing with the immediate first aid usually requires brief rest, support, and ice to control inflammation. More serious injuries may need emergency medical attention.

Many professional athletes have benefited from Matrix Repatterning. Injuries that used to be career ending may now potentially be resolved using these breakthrough technologies.

It is important to remember that injuries exist against a background of all previous injuries and the resulting patterns of tension arising from those events. In other words, your strained knee may need your immediate attention; however, the hip you fell on last winter and the ankle you strained three summers ago may be the reason the knee was vulnerable to the most recent injury and the reason it continues to resist attempts to resolve the situation.

With this in mind, it would be an excellent idea to perform a self-assessment and self-treatment (see chapter 4) of the entire body as part of your conditioning program and in order to prevent injury. This would go a long way toward balancing the tensions in the body and establishing a high level of resilience and tolerance to excessive force in whatever activity you engage in. I believe this would prevent many injuries from having any significant effect on the body.

Many professional athletes have benefited from treatment using Matrix Repatterning. Injuries that used to be career ending may now potentially be resolved using these breakthrough technologies.

Mark's Story: An Athlete Finds a Second Lease on Life

I was contacted by a chiropractor working in a large sports medicine facility. He had heard of my work, and because he was frustrated with a particular case, he called to find out if I would see Mark, a decathlete. I agreed to see him for a consultation. In reviewing Mark's history, I found he had encountered repeated straining injuries to his knees and thigh and groin muscles. Despite extensive treatment using state-of-the-art methods, he was not progressing.

In my examination I found that his thigh muscles and hip muscles were seriously imbalanced. Indeed, the other members of his treatment team had found the same problem and had valiantly tried to stretch and goad these muscles into some semblance of symmetry. Unfortunately, they were all unsuccessful.

I found that his primary restrictions were in his hip and thighbones and proceeded to release these tension patterns. With one treatment I was able to restore the muscles of his hips and thighs back into balance. Since then Mark has progressed significantly and with a few more treatments was able to fully re-enter his training program and is now preparing for the Olympics.

I believe Mark's case clearly illustrates some of the erroneous assumptions made with regard to so-called "sports injuries." Many clinics and clinicians are eagerly tackling the perceived muscle imbalances, including what they call torn muscles and ligaments, since these areas are, of course, the site of symptoms. Hundreds of thousands of dollars and countless hours (and many careers) are sacrificed each year on ineffective treatments, not only in the field of athletics, but in many areas of physical medicine. This is not to suggest that the other forms of treatment and the training regimes are of no value, but that when applied without a full appraisal of the primary sources of imbalance, they are often less effective than anticipated. My clinical experience has shown that Matrix Repatterning, along with a sound program of exercise therapy, can form the basis of a powerful set of tools to help athletes back into ideal biomechanical efficiency and optimal performance. For more information about some helpful exercise measures to help support the effectiveness of Matrix Repatterning, please see chapter 8.

MOTOR VEHICLE COLLISIONS

We now have more people driving more places in more cars at higher speeds. The result is people in cars meeting other people in cars with more force of impact, more often. And more often than not, everyone involved is feeling the effects of these encounters for a lot longer than they would like to.

Much effort and energy has gone into trying to measure and quantify the effects of motor vehicle collisions on the spine, including the neck, but as it turns out, these efforts have not borne much fruit. As you may have already read in the section above on the spine, these joints and tissues were brilliantly designed to *give* with force and apparently have tremendous tolerance to the bending and twisting that occurs in most injuries.

It's amazing how much force it actually takes to damage these tissues. This is not to say that primary injury of the spine is not possible or that is doesn't occur. It is only to suggest that in most cases, the actual production of primary restrictions within the spine itself is quite rare.

Several studies have demonstrated that a much more common occurrence in the types of impact common in motor vehicle collisions is indirect trauma to the large, fluid-filled organs in the chest and abdomen. Lacerations and actual rupture (bursting) of these organs is common in severe impacts. These injuries can often be life threatening (NIH 1985; Fingerhut 1997).

What is less well-recognized are the more common, less critical injuries to these organs that occur in more moderate impacts. In these cases, the organs expand on impact and become rigid. They develop primary restrictions and exert a powerful influence on the entire structure, distorting the spine and many other musculoskeletal structures, causing painful strain patterns.

These effects tend to be overlooked because they do not show up on X-rays or other forms of imaging, nor do they necessarily result in gross disease states that are detectable from blood or urine tests. However, with the Matrix Repatterning assessment, their influence is obvious. Treatment of these primary restrictions often results in rapid resolution of many painful conditions and the restoration of normal, pain-free ranges of motion.

Other common injuries include head trauma and impact or fracture of the arms or legs. Matrix Repatterning, due its facility in precisely locating the pattern of injury in bone, is able to address these aspects of motor vehicle collisions very efficiently. Head injuries are discussed in some detail later in this chapter.

FIBROMYALGIA: IT JUST HURTS EVERYWHERE

Fibromyalgia or fibromyalgia syndrome is a widespread musculoskeletal pain and fatigue disorder for which the cause is still unknown. *Fibromyalgia* means pain in the muscles, ligaments, and tendons—the soft, fibrous tissues in the body. Most patients with fibromyalgia say that they ache all over. Their muscles may feel like they have been pulled or overworked. Sometimes the muscles twitch, and at other times they burn. More women than men are afflicted with fibromyalgia, and it occurs in all age groups.

Some describe the symptoms as being like the muscle aches and pains associated with the flu. There is also an associated loss of energy and another condition, chronic fatigue syndrome, is sometimes associated with fibromyalgia. Sleep disturbances, depression, irritable bowel syndrome, and TMJ syndrome (pain in the jaw) also appear to be associated with the disorder. Other common symptoms include cognitive or memory impairment, premenstrual syndrome, painful menstrual periods, chest pain, morning stiffness, numbness and tingling sensations, muscle twitching, irritable bladder, skin sensitivities, dry eyes and mouth, dizziness, and impaired coordination. Patients are often sensitive to foods, chemicals, odors, loud noise, and bright light.

The origins of this condition have eluded researchers ever since it was first defined. The term itself is essentially meaningless: *algia* meaning pain; *fibro* and *myo* referring to the location of the pain in the fibrous tissues and the muscles, which are everywhere! It is associated with many things (including viruses, stress, injuries, depression, sleep disturbance, brain chemistry and hormonal imbalances, and chemical and heavy metal toxicity) and nothing in particular. As such, it is a source of frustration for the sufferer and the health-care practitioner alike.

Matrix Repatterning may offer some insights and some possible hope. Many common impact injuries, including falls and motor vehicle accidents, have been associated with the onset of fibromyalgia. In previous chapters, the mechanism of injury at the cellular/molecular level was discussed. The tensegrity matrix could explain some of the widespread mechanical effects of certain more serious injuries. One or more primary sites of restriction may be the source of strain and pain throughout the body due to the interconnected nature of the matrix. Also, the deeper underlying issues of bone and fluid-filled organ involvement could explain why many of these conditions have gone unresolved.

As explained earlier, these types of injuries have significant effects on the structure and function of certain internal organs. The heart, liver, kidneys, and spleen are particularly vulnerable to the effects of impact, and indications are that their physiology is altered when the cells are under abnormal tension. The liver, for example, regulates many of the hormones and chemicals in the body, as well as functioning to rid the body of toxic materials. If it is impaired by trauma, the levels of these substances might well become abnormal. This could be one possible cause of the chemical imbalances associated with fibromyalgia (Waylonis and Perkins 1994).

My experience treating fibromyalgia and related conditions has been promising. Resolving the structural component of the layers of injury present has often opened a window, allowing the light of deeper healing to occur. The body, once restored to structural and mechanical balance, functions more efficiently and with less strain. One of the most common statements by patients with fibromyalgia upon resolving some of these issues with Matrix Repatterning is that their sleep patterns are restored to normal. It is my opinion that the background of irritation from primary restrictions and their resulting strain patterns is a constant source of neurological "noise," leading to a heightened state of alarm within the nervous system. Once these sources of irritability are reduced, the patient often experiences a welcome relief, as if the volume of noise had been turned down dramatically. Clinical experience has also shown promise in the restoration of normal organ function, which could lead to a normalization of hormonal levels and improved digestive and detoxification systems. The exercise program outlined in chapter 8 may also assist in the restoration of flexibility, strength, and general fitness levels in these cases.

Evelyn's Story: Easing the Pain of Fibromyalgia

Evelyn looked defeated as she sat down in front of me to begin our consultation. She had just reluctantly been given the diagnosis she had suspected and feared. She had been harassing her doctor to acknowledge her pain and had spent a considerable amount of time researching her own condition. She had come to the opinion some months earlier that she might have fibromyalgia, but she could not get her doctor to budge on his reluctance to acknowledge her suspicions. Finally, after numerous tests, he finally gave in and confirmed her suspicions. She did indeed have the dread disease. Why, she asked him, had he not made the diagnosis earlier, given the overwhelming evidence from her symptoms alone. He admitted that he had been reluctant to do so, since telling her she definitely had fibromyalgia meant that he would have to give up on her, since there was no cure.

Evelyn then came to see me on the insistence of her sister, whom I had helped following a serious car accident. She had told Evelyn how all the doctors had given up on her as well, with her constant back and neck pain and recurring dizzy spells. She had explained how I had been able to discover the primary sources of tension in her internal organs, spine, and head and how I had easily been able to release these so that she had begun to experience almost immediate relief after nearly two years of life-altering pain.

Despite her sister's enthusiasm, Evelyn could not seem to muster much in the way of hope for herself. She had been given the bad news that she was now a statistic, and the statistics for fibromyalgia were none too optimistic.

So, here she was, victorious in proving that she had a real condition—justification for all the pain she had endured—and defeated by the pronouncement that her doctor, and indeed medicine, had no answers.

I explained the premise behind Matrix Repatterning, how structural imbalance could contribute to strain and pain, and how studies had shown that cellular tension could produce changes in the way cells function and process chemicals. In fact, due to their high fluid content, many of the internal organs were extremely vulnerable to impact injuries from falls and car accidents.

Evelyn suddenly got a very thoughtful look on her face. "I had a fall off a ladder about two years ago. Do you think there might be a connection?"

"When did you start to have pain?" I asked.

"I had some aches and pains for a while after the fall, but I didn't think much about it. Then about a year and a half ago, I got a bad case of flu. Right after that, everything started to hurt all the time."

"Mmm," I pondered. "The timing could be right. Let's go ahead and see what your body has to say, since everything is recorded there." I directed Evelyn to the examination area and began my assessment.

When I was finished, I had found several primary restrictions in the pelvis and some of the internal organs, which correlated with the fall off the ladder she had described. I also found evidence of a head injury, which she recalled experiencing in a bicycle accident when she was twelve. I explained that the nature and extent of her injuries could account for much of her pain, and that the injuries to her internal organs, specifically her liver, could be part of the reason for the chemical imbalance, reducing her pain tolerance.

I noticed that Evelyn's face suddenly seemed brighter. She indicated to me that she was interested in getting started right away in resolving the issues I had uncovered. I had her schedule a series of appointments. I also suggested she sign up for one of our ongoing self-treatment classes, where she could learn to handle some of her own pain. I explained that she would learn some basic first-aid Matrix Repatterning techniques as well as stretching and toning exercises to increase her flexibility and fitness level.

Within six weeks, Evelyn was a different person. She had discovered that there was indeed a cause for her pain and that addressing it at this level paid enormous dividends. Not only was she practically free of pain, she was becoming more fit than ever and, more importantly, she had retaken control of her health and her life.

REPETITIVE STRAIN INJURY

The assembly-line worker and the secretary now have something in common. When they have pain on the job, they are often given the same diagnosis. Any job that involves repetitive motion, whether it involves turning a wrench on a car part or using a computer keyboard, may lead to pain in various areas of the body. Carpal tunnel syndrome, neck and back strain, headache, foot or leg pain, and many other symptoms have been attributed to a condition variously called repetitive injury syndrome, repetitive strain disorder, or cumulative trauma disorder.

The problem with this type of diagnosis is that it is apparently unpredictable with regard to who may be affected or not. There may be ten or more employees performing the same operation on an assembly line. One might develop shoulder and arm pain, another might have low back pain, while a third might experience knee pain. The other seven may experience no symptoms whatsoever. So, are these problems due to the activities on the job? If that were the case, you would expect each of the workers to have similar types of symptoms. So, what's the real problem here?

It has been the experience of many Matrix Repatterning practitioners that when the underlying primary restrictions are resolved, many of these so-called repetitive injuries simply disappear. In many of those cases, the area of symptoms (pain) was not the primary area requiring treatment.

Let us examine this finding in the light of what we know about the nature of the tensegrity matrix. In the case where there is a true molecular shift (primary restrictions), some activities that would normally be well tolerated and perhaps produce only a temporary strain could now lead to an aggravation of the pre-existing problem. This is because the area of primary molecular restriction is unable to dissipate the forces of any activity as efficiently as healthy tissue. Moderate amounts of force may cause additional molecules around the original primary area of involvement to become affected. Repetitive movement, especially accompanied by a load (weight or resistance), may accentuate the restriction already present within the area.

This means that a part of the body that is not moving properly or has lost some of its flexibility will tend to absorb more of the force of certain activities without being able to release the build-up in tension or resistance. As the individual attempts to perform the activity, the patterns of strain will be accentuated throughout the body, causing abnormal motion in many other areas as they are required to move in compensation for the area(s) of primary restriction. Therefore, what another individual might experience as a minor strain, easily resolved after a brief rest period, would for a person with abnormal patterns of restriction within their structure, lead to an increase in the tendency to overload sensitive joint, muscle, and fascial tissues. Eventually, it would require less and less strain or time at the activity to produce inflammation and pain.

The solution, of course, is to address the true sources of the mechanical imbalances within the body. Matrix Repatterning offers a significant tool to be able to detect and resolve these conditions at this most fundamental level, painlessly and often permanently. The self-treatment methods described in this book may address many of these issues; however, complex problems may require the intervention of a trained professional.

HEAD INJURIES: THEY'RE ALL IN YOUR HEAD

The cranium is that part of the head that forms a protective container for the brain. Direct injuries to the head are very common and can occur beginning at a very young age. The inside of the head is actually mostly water in the form of a substance called *cerebrospinal fluid*, which surrounds and forms most of the mass of the brain itself. Water, as we know, is a very dense and heavy substance. The fact that our head is located way up on top of our two-legged body makes it a likely candidate for injuries when we fall. Injuries occurring during contact sports, motor vehicle collisions, and occupational incidents are also common.

The outer covering of the brain is composed of thick, fibrous layers of fascia called the *meninges*, as well as a thin layer of bone. The bony plates making up the skull are connected in several places by long, zigzagging joints called *sutures*. There are also several fibrous reinforcing membranes in and around the brain, which are attached to the outer wall.

Impact injuries to the head create fluid shock waves that can have a significant effect on the structure of the cranium and the brain itself. This is often referred to as a concussion. When an injury occurs, the shock waves travel from the point of impact to the opposite side of the cranium. This creates a pushing in of the head at the site of impact and an outward bulging on the opposite side. Injury forces, if significant, will cause a permanent reaction at the molecular level. Depending on the direction of the impact, certain joints and other elements of the head may also become strained and locked in various ways.

One of the reasons for the wide-ranging effects of head injury is the fact that the membranes surrounding the brain (the meninges), like the entire tensegrity matrix, are able to conduct electricity. The brain is made up of nerves, which produce electrical impulses. When a distortion occurs in the meninges, its ability to conduct electricity changes. These areas of altered conductivity could conceivably become potential short circuits in the transmission of impulses generated by the brain.

This may be the reason that head injury is associated with so many conditions, including headache, ringing in the ears (tinnitus), dizziness (vertigo), seizure disorders like epilepsy and narcolepsy, sensory and motor disorders, speech pathology, visual problems, and cognitive and learning disorders. These conditions are very common and many unsuspected cranial injuries may be responsible for these conditions.

New research from the University of Warwick reveals that children with even mild head injury may be at risk of long-term complications, including personality changes and emotional, behavioral, and learning problems (Hawley 2004).

■ Ted's Story: Shrinking the Problem

It was the end of the day and I was preparing to shut down the clinic for the weekend when the phone rang. The woman's voice was strained, yet cordial. She had heard about me from a friend and wondered if I could help her husband. Ted was in severe distress with neck and shoulder pain. She was politely insistent that I see him on an emergency basis, and sensing her distress, I agreed.

Later that afternoon, Ted and his wife, Helen, arrived at my office. He was a large man of fifty-five with a distinguished beard and a jovial if somewhat strained demeanor. I noticed that he had a large scar on his forehead. I proceeded to examine him and noticed that one of the major primary areas of tension appeared in the back of his head. I palpated the area to discover a lump the size of half a grapefruit on the left side of his head. I asked him about head injuries, and he mentioned a motorcycle accident in which his head had struck the pavement with such force that his helmet had shattered. He had, since that injury, suffered from increasingly severe headaches, to the point that now he had pain twenty-four hours a day and could not sleep for more than half an hour at a time without awakening in pain.

I explained how forces are transmitted through the skull. The part of the skull around the brain is essentially a fluid-filled structure surrounded by hard bone. Impact injuries can create changes in the bone structure in the area of impact, sometimes appearing as flattened areas or dents. The force may then be transmitted by the fluid inside the head, causing areas on the opposite side to expand outward. This could account for the large bulge I had noticed. I also indicated that the problem in his skull was influencing his entire body and that, despite the fact that his pain was in his neck and shoulder, one of the primary sources of tension was in his head. He was a retired science teacher. The theory made sense to him, and he agreed to allow me to treat his head.

I proceeded to apply gentle pressure at the center of tension located in his skull. Within a few minutes, I began to feel the typical pattern of release as the tissues under my hands began to soften. I had experienced this phenomenon countless times before and had witnessed significant structural and shape changes in bones, muscles, ligaments, and heads. But this was a very large bulge. I didn't expect any miracles. Well, to my surprise, that massive lump completely dissolved under my fingertips.

At first, I could not believe it. This thing was huge! And now it was gone!

I sat in stunned silence for several minutes, continuing to feel his now normal-shaped skull. I finally asked Ted to reach up to the back of his head and feel for himself. His comment was: "What did you do? Where is the lump?" Well, that was the confirmation I needed to decide that at least I wasn't losing my mind. I asked him how he felt. He stated that he felt quite relaxed and that his head felt much more comfortable. When he got off the table, he noticed that his neck and shoulders were freer and less painful.

When I saw him next, about two weeks later, he told me his neck and shoulders had been fine and that the lump in his head was still completely gone. He had no more headaches, and he was sleeping like a baby right through the night for the first time in years.

TOOTH OR CONSEQUENCES: DENTAL ISSUES

The tooth is a unique structure in that it is the only part of the skeleton that is exposed. This extremely dense structure is capable of withstanding the tremendous forces of chewing and, with reasonable care, is designed to last a lifetime of grinding and compression. Direct facial impact often results in dental lesions. Falls, motor vehicle collisions, and sports injuries are common, and these kinds of incidents can produce lasting strain patterns in and around the teeth.

One fact of modern life in the past one hundred or so years is the advent of technology in the field of dentistry. Dental extraction can be a particularly traumatic procedure that may produce significant tissue trauma and scar tissue. There is another, seemingly innocuous procedure that has gone unnoticed as a potential source of dental trauma. The modern, high-speed drill is capable of introducing a powerful vibration—a form of mechanical energy—directly into the highly dense tissues that make up the teeth as well as the surrounding bone in which they are embedded. This energy is, in my opinion, the source of a significant proportion of the primary dental lesions found increasingly by Matrix Repatterning practitioners.

The fact that these lesions are so common despite the absence of an obvious history of trauma was my first clue that some other mechanism must be at the root (no pun intended) of this source of dysfunction. It is my belief that the mechanical force from the drill is converted by the molecular structure of the tissues in such a way as to alter the molecular relationships within the tensegrity structure. The net effect is that a strain pattern is produced similar to that seen with any other injuries.

Jim's Story: Out of Commission

Jim Booth, a local dentist and a good friend, called at the end of my workday. His usually jovial demeanor seemed a tad strained. He explained that his arm had become increasingly numb and weak over the past few days. He had been able to stretch it out and restore it to a relatively normal state until today. Now it was completely paralyzed! I checked to make sure I had heard him right. I had. I didn't know what to say. I told him to get to my office as soon as he could.

I had seen Jim several times over the years for many sports-related injuries. He was quite the daredevil—barefoot water-skiing and boating were his favorite pursuits. But now his arm was paralyzed. I could sense the fear in his voice. His whole livelihood depended on his hands. My mind began racing over a possible diagnosis. I was not optimistic.

I greeted him at the door. His smile was strained, and I noticed the fine layer of perspiration on his face. He had canceled his entire workday due to his infirmity. We went into my consultation room. I asked him if he had had an injury. He said he hadn't. I proceeded to examine him, hoping for the best.

I noticed that he had a significant amount of spasm in the muscles extending from the front of his neck on the left. These muscles can sometimes press on the nerves going from the neck to the arm. I found that the muscles in his left arm were practically useless, and none of his normal reflexes were present.

I used my usual procedure to determine the primary restriction but came up with nothing significant. I asked him again if he had injured himself in any way. He told me again that he hadn't. Then he thought about it and mentioned that he had just had a tooth extracted by a colleague of his the week before.

Well, I thought, I had nothing to lose. I placed my hand over the side of his face where the tooth had been extracted. Bingo! The muscles in his neck relaxed profoundly. I put on a latex glove and proceeded to release the tension within the tooth socket with gentle pressure applied in a particular way. Within minutes, the feeling in his arm and hand returned. By the time he left, he had regained full use.

At the time it seemed ironic to me that this momentous discovery about the influence of the teeth on the rest of the body should have been have been revealed to me while working with a dentist. But, then again, life is interesting!

SCAR TISSUE: MAKING THE BEST OF A BAD SITUATION

Scar tissue is part of the repair process, one of the ways the body responds in the face of tissue damage or loss of tissue. Cuts, burns, fractures, severe infections, inflammation (due to any source of significant irritation), or surgery may result in the laying down of varying degrees of fibrous tissue strands called *scar tissue*. This is the body's way of attempting to restore tissue integrity and protect against further injury or infection. The laying down of scar tissue—also referred to as *adhesions*—is in direct proportion to the degree of the tissue trauma and the background condition of the individual. The latter may be influenced by general health, including pre-existing autoimmune and inflammatory conditions, as well as genetic factors.

Scar tissue is a compromise in that it may save your life, but there is always a cost. The cost is the increased tension at the site of the scar. This is why scar tissue often appears as a primary restriction in the Matrix Repatterning assessment of the body. Scar tissue is treatable; however it may not be possible to restore it to completely normal function once it has formed. Therapy is directed to reduce restriction, to encourage the body to reabsorb as much of the excess fibrous material as possible, and ultimately to restore normal or near-normal tissue compliance and elasticity.

This is why I refer to the treatment of scar tissue as making the best of a bad situation. Fortunately, in most cases, taking care of many of the other sources of primary restriction in other tissues, such as organs, bones, and joints, produces so much improvement in overall function that the relative influence of persisting scars can be minimized. Matrix Repatterning practitioners often use microcurrent therapy in addition to their hands-on treatments. Microcurrent therapy has been found to greatly assist the possibilities of normalizing and reducing the effects of scar tissue (Biedebach 1989; Doubler 1994). Certain self-treatment measures can also support the maintenance of these areas in a functional state (see "Castor Oil Compress" in appendix 2).

FRACTURES AS "CRUMPLE ZONES"

I refer to fractures as "crumple zones" since I see them as similar reactions to trauma as the front and rear ends of some cars in a collision. Crumple zones are designed to absorb the force of an injury and thus protect more vital tissues from injury. Most of us think of fractures as a bad thing, and certainly no one likes to get hurt or be in pain. However, considering the lasting damage certain injuries could inflict, sometimes getting away with just a broken bone may be a blessing in disguise.

Have you ever heard it said that a serious strain or sprain is worse than a broken bone? In many cases, this may be very true. In a fracture, the incoming force of the injury actually severs the glue that holds the molecules together. Remember, under normal circumstances the force of an injury travels throughout the body due to the *continuous* nature of the tensegrity matrix.

Guess what happens when the matrix is suddenly no longer continuous? That's right, the force cannot go any further and *voila!*—the injury is stopped dead in its tracks. This is the same idea as employing a back burn to contain a forest fire. This is where another controlled fire is created along the track of the fire that is out of control. When the fire reaches the already burned-out area it dies, since there is no fuel for it to progress.

The main concern with fractures is the strain to the ligaments and muscles, as well as the bones that absorbed the force of the injury. If, for example, you fell on your arm and it resulted in a fracture of the forearm, the molecules in the parts of the bone nearest the hand and wrist would be most affected by the force of impact. The energy of the injury tends to be dissipated as it is absorbed by the parts of the body in direct contact with the incoming force. As mentioned previously, certain internal organs may also be injured if an impact was involved.

Unfortunately, modern medicine tends to concern itself only with things that show up on conventional tests, such as the X-ray. Soft-tissue injuries (affecting the muscles, ligaments, joints, and the internal organs, as well as the molecular restrictions within bone) do not show up on X-rays, and so are usually discounted. In reality, it is many of these aspects of the injury that continue to plague the sufferer and may cause ongoing problems and even serious complications.

Dianne's Story: An Arm Restored

Dianne was an Olympic-rowing hopeful. She was a pleasant, very positive, albeit frustrated young lady of twenty when I met her. She had suffered a freak accident while climbing and had fractured her left humerus (the bone of the upper arm). Weeks and months went by. Her doctors X-rayed her arm after a routine casting of six weeks. The fracture had not healed at all. Further casting for another month proved futile as well. She was then referred to an orthopedic surgeon, and a procedure was performed to attach the two portions of bone using a metal plate and six screws. Two years later, she still had no union of the bones.

When she was finally referred to me, it was two and a half years after the original injury. The bones had still not fused, and her left arm was essentially a useless appendage, hanging at her side. I examined her and found I could literally slide the two portions of the bone backward, forward, and side to side, all while hearing the sickening scraping sound this movement made. Even with the dramatic results of this maneuver, Dianne felt no pain. It was positively eerie.

Based on her previous experience, Dianne didn't have high expectations, but she realized that conventional medicine had no more to offer her. The thought of more surgery with very little promise of success made her cringe. She had pleaded with her doctor to look into other possibilities. That was when she discovered my work, while conferring with a physical therapist who had heard of me.

I told Dianne what I tell all of my patients, and it is what I encourage my students to tell their patients: "I am not concerned with your symptoms." In Dianne's case I also added that I was not concerned with her fracture. My one and only goal was to release the structural imbalances present in her body in order to allow the body to normalize and to support its self-healing ability.

This point is very important since it removes the mysticism from the healing process. The doctor or practitioner is not the healer. The body always heals itself. If anything, the practitioner is simply a facilitator of the healing process. I strongly believe that this allows the patient and practitioner to enter into a healthier relationship, where both work together to support the process.

I treated Dianne four times over a two-month period. My treatment focused on releasing all sources of primary tension throughout her body related to all of the accumulated injuries she had experienced. Due to the deteriorated condition of the bone, I also utilized microcurrent electrotherapy, which I find to greatly facilitate the healing process by normalizing the electrical field in severely injured tissue.

After one month Dianne and I both noticed that her arm was becoming stronger and that I could no longer move the bones across each other. When she was re-examined after three months, her doctor announced that the bones had fused significantly. She continued to progress, and her arm completely healed within six months.

Matrix Repatterning practitioners rely entirely on the body tissues to direct where the treatment needs to be performed, and this largely frees them from the tyranny of symptoms and the often misleading focus on a particular diagnosis. The idea that Dianne's problem was solely located at the fracture site is an extremely limiting concept based on the body functioning as separate parts. The tensegrity matrix is a continuous fabric, which means that tension arising from anywhere in the body could be a factor in limiting functional integrity and the healing process elsewhere in the body. Dianne's story illustrates the power of the body to heal itself. The lesson learned: Get rid of anything interfering with the normal functioning of the body and get out of the way. Let the body do it!

Matrix Repatterning has the potential to help restore structural balance to the entire body. Medical research is beginning to reveal the mechanical and structural aspects of many conditions (Ingber 1998, 2002; Pollack 2001). Evidence is mounting that a disturbance of the matrix at the cellular level may play a role in many health issues. The accounts in this chapter represent a very brief overview of the types of conditions that appear to respond to Matrix Repatterning. We are hopeful that our ongoing research will broaden our understanding of this marvelous machine known as the human body, and open new and exciting horizons in helping us achieve and maintain optimal health and well-being.

CHAPTER 7

Quick Reference Guide for Specific Conditions

This chapter covers a number of common areas of the body amenable to treatment using Matrix Repatterning. It is important to remember that pain in one part of the body may be a symptom of a larger pattern of tension arising from sources anywhere in the body. The treatment program is designed to help you zero in on some of the more common areas that may be producing a particular problem. If your condition does not respond favorably within one or two sessions, refer back to the general guidelines for scanning the entire body.

Be aware that any condition may be due to any primary source of restriction anywhere in the body. Remember that the teeth and the spine are potential sources of symptoms over a wide range of possibilities because of their nerve and reflex connections. In general, the neck and upper spine may cause symptoms in the upper half of the body, while the lower spine and pelvis are associated with symptoms in the lower half. Similarly, the upper teeth may be related to symptoms from the waist up and the lower teeth may cause symptoms from the waist down.

The following are covered in this section: headache, jaw pain, neck pain, shoulder pain, elbow pain, hand and wrist pain, upper back pain, low back pain, hip pain, knee pain, and foot and ankle pain.

Note: It is strongly recommended that you seek professional advice if pain comes on suddenly without any history of injury, is worse at night, or does not respond to self-treatment within a reasonable amount of time, or worsens.

HOW TO USE THE TREATMENT TABLES

Conditions or areas of the body where your pain may be located are listed in this section from the head down. Locate the chart that is closest to the one that describes your symptoms. Named conditions such as "tennis elbow" are often arbitrary, and any pain in the elbow could be associated with the primary restrictions listed for that condition. Follow the steps below:

1. Test the resistance of the indicator (thigh muscle, fingers, or thumb) without placing your other hand on any other part of your body. Then keep that hand on the indicator without pushing on it.
2. Place your other hand on one of the locations from the list in the second column (common primary restrictions).
3. Test the indicator by pushing on the thigh muscle or on the fingers or thumb. See if there is an increased give or softening of the indicator.
4. Test the next area on the list of common primary restrictions.
5. Determine which of the areas you tested is the most significant, based on the degree of give produced in the indicator. The area that causes the greatest amount of give or softening of the indicator is the most significant primary restriction.
6. Treat the primary restriction according to the instructions under the treatment column.
7. Treat any other primary restrictions that you found from the list of common primary restrictions.

Matrix Repatterning is designed to restore structural balance to the body. Pain is often the result of strain in areas of the body that have been compensating for the primary restrictions. As a result, inflammation may have developed over a period of time, leading to the accumulation of pain-producing chemical changes. The nerve supply to the area of pain may become irritated and inflamed as well. For these reasons, the pain you are experiencing may take a period of time to resolve as the tissues re-establish a more normal, balanced state. In certain cases, you may also experience some increase in discomfort in other areas for one to three days following treatment. This may be due to a reawakening of pain signals that the nervous system had adapted to previously. It is recommended that you refrain from vigorous physical activity and drink additional water for twenty-four to forty-eight hours after treatment. Epsom salt baths or castor oil packs may also be helpful (see appendix 2).

Condition: Headache			
Description	**Common Primary Restrictions**	**Quick Tests**	**Treatment**
Headaches may be localized in one area, they may be generalized, or they may move around. They may be related to structural imbalance, disease, or stress. Any headache that does not respond to self-treatment or becomes worse should be investigated by a health professional.	■ Head ■ Jaw ■ Teeth ■ Neck	Head: Top, forehead, sides, back Jaw: Upper jaw, lower jaw Teeth: Upper teeth, lower teeth Neck: Back of neck, throat	Head, jaws, teeth: Place the hand over the area indicated and leave in place until release is felt. Neck: Place the hand over the area indicated and leave in place until release is felt. Alternatively, while holding your hand over the area, bend the head forward, backward, and sideways, and rotate to the left and the right. Hold in the position creating the greatest softening of the indicator until release is felt.

Condition: Jaw Pain (TMJ)			
Description	**Common Primary Restrictions**	**Quick Tests**	**Treatment**
Pain in the jaw may be experienced during chewing or talking. It may be due to local inflammation and structural imbalance or due to tension arising from other areas creating abnormal movement and strain of the jaw joint. Dental misalignment is often blamed for this problem; however it is often the result of a larger imbalance, including the jaw itself.	■ Head ■ Jaws ■ Teeth ■ Neck	<u>Head:</u> Top, forehead, sides, back <u>Jaw:</u> Upper jaw, lower jaw <u>Teeth:</u> Upper teeth, lower teeth <u>Neck:</u> Back of neck, throat	<u>Head, jaws, teeth:</u> Place your hand over the area indicated and leave in place until release is felt. <u>Neck:</u> Place your hand over the area indicated and leave in place until release is felt. Alternatively, while holding your hand over the area, bend the head forward, backward, and sideways, and rotate to the left and the right. Hold in the position creating the greatest softening of the indicator until release is felt.

Condition: Neck Pain			
Description	**Common Primary Restrictions**	**Quick Tests**	**Treatment**
Pain located in the neck area may be aggravated by certain activities such as moving the head or arms. Pain in the neck may be due to local structural imbalance or to other sources of tension arising from the chest (including organ lesions), shoulders, or from a tooth. This area is also a common area for tension due to stress. Neck pain that arises without any obvious strain or that doesn't respond to self-treatment should be investigated by a health professional.	■ Neck ■ Chest ■ Shoulder ■ Teeth	Neck: Back of neck, throat Chest: Front of chest (use palm of hand), back of chest (use back of hand), sides of chest Shoulder: Front, side, and back of shoulder Teeth: Upper teeth, lower teeth	Neck: Place your hand over the area indicated and leave in place until release is felt. Alternatively, while holding the hand over the area, bend the head forward, backward, and sideways, and rotate to the left and the right. Hold in the position creating the greatest softening of the indicator until release is felt. Shoulder: Place the hand over the area indicated and leave in place until release is felt. Alternatively, move the shoulder joint in the direction creating the greatest softening of the indicator and hold until release is felt. Chest, teeth: Place the hand over the area indicated and leave in place until release is felt.

Condition: Shoulder Pain			
Description	**Common Primary Restrictions**	**Quick Tests**	**Treatment**
Shoulder pain may be due to local structural problems or from tension arising in surrounding areas. Pain due to structural imbalance is usually aggravated by movement. The shoulder may also be painful due to other disease processes. Any shoulder pain that is not affected by movement or position or does not respond to self-treatment should be investigated by a health professional.	■ Shoulder ■ Upper arm ■ Neck ■ Chest ■ Upper Teeth	Shoulder: Front, side, and back of shoulder Upper arm: Upper, middle, and lower part of upper arm Neck: Back of neck, throat Chest: Front of chest (use palm of hand), back of chest (use back of hand), sides of chest Upper Teeth: Upper teeth	Shoulder, arm, chest, upper teeth: Place the hand over the area indicated and leave in place until release is felt. Alternatively, move the shoulder joint and upper arm bone in the direction creating the greatest softening of the indicator and hold until release is felt. Neck: Place the hand over the area indicated and leave in place until release is felt. Alternatively, while holding your hand over the area, bend the head forward, backward, and sideways, and rotate to the left and the right. Hold in the position creating the greatest softening of the indicator until release is felt.

Condition: Elbow Pain			
Description	**Common Primary Restrictions**	**Quick Tests**	**Treatment**
Elbow pain may be due to local structural problems or from tension arising in surrounding areas. Pain due to structural imbalance is usually aggravated by movement. Tennis elbow and golfer's elbow are painful conditions of the tendons and muscles crossing the elbow joint. They may be referred to as *epicondylitis* or *tendonitis* of the elbow. So-called tennis elbow involves the outside of the elbow, while golfer's elbow occurs on the inside of the elbow. These conditions can occur in people who are not involved in either of the sports that give these conditions their names.	■ Elbow ■ Upper arm ■ Forearm ■ Neck ■ Chest ■ Upper Teeth	Elbow: Front and back of elbow Arm or forearm: Upper, middle, and lower arm, upper, middle, and lower forearm Neck: Back of neck, throat Chest: Front of chest (use palm of hand), back of chest (use back of hand), sides of chest Upper teeth: Upper teeth	Elbow, arm, forearm, chest, upper teeth: Place the hand over the area indicated and leave in place until release is felt. Alternatively, move the elbow joint, arm, and forearm bones in the direction creating the greatest softening of the indicator and hold until release is felt. Neck: Place your hand over the area indicated and leave in place until release is felt. Alternatively, while holding the hand over the area, bend the head forward, backward, and sideways, and rotate to the left and the right. Hold in the position creating the greatest softening of the indicator until release is felt.

Condition: Hand and Wrist Pain			
Description	**Common Primary Restrictions**	**Quick Tests**	**Treatment**
Pain in the hand and wrist may arise due to a straining injury, an impact, or various sports- and work-related injuries. Pain may be accompanied by swelling and may be aggravated by certain movements. Upper limb pain may also arise from a primary restriction in the elbow, forearm, chest, upper back, neck, or teeth. Carpal tunnel syndrome is characterized by numbness, tingling, pain, burning, stiffness, or swelling in one or both hands. It may be aggravated by certain activities or positions.	■ Hand ■ Wrist ■ Forearm ■ Chest ■ Neck ■ Upper teeth	Hand, wrist: Front and back of hand and wrist Forearm: Upper, middle, and lower forearm Chest: Front of chest (use palm of hand), back of chest (use back of hand), sides of chest Neck: Back of neck, throat Upper teeth: Upper teeth	Hand, wrist, forearm, chest, upper teeth: Place the hand over the area indicated and leave in place until release is felt. Alternatively, move the hand and wrist joints and the forearm bones in the direction creating the greatest softening of the indicator and hold until release is felt. Neck: Place the hand over the area indicated and leave in place until release is felt. Alternatively, while holding the hand over the area, bend the head forward, backward, and sideways, and rotate to the left and the right. Hold in the position creating the greatest softening of the indicator until release is felt.

Condition: Upper Back Pain			
Description	**Common Primary Restrictions**	**Quick Tests**	**Treatment**
Pain located in the spinal area may be aggravated by certain activities such as lifting, bending, twisting, walking, or other forms of strenuous activity. Back pain that arises without any obvious strain or does not respond to self-treatment should be investigated by a health professional.	■ Chest ■ Upper back ■ Shoulder ■ Upper teeth	Chest, upper back: Front of chest (use palm of hand), back of chest (use back of hand), sides of chest Shoulder: Front, side, and back of shoulder Upper teeth: Upper teeth	Shoulder: Place the hand over the area indicated and leave in place until release is felt. Alternatively, move the shoulder joint and arm bone in the direction creating the greatest softening of the indicator and hold until release is felt. Upper back: While holding the hand over the area of the chest indicated, feel for the greatest softening of the indicator until release is felt. Chest, upper teeth: Place the hand over the area indicated and leave in place until release is felt.

Condition: Low Back Pain			
Description	**Common Primary Restrictions**	**Quick Tests**	**Treatment**
Pain located in the spinal area may be aggravated by certain activities such as lifting, bending, twisting, walking, or other forms of strenuous activity. Back pain that arises without any obvious strain or does not respond to self-treatment should be investigated by a health professional.	■ Pelvis ■ Lower back ■ Abdomen ■ Hips ■ Lower teeth	<u>Pelvis:</u> Side, front, and back of pelvis <u>Lower back, abdomen:</u> Front of abdomen (use palm of hand), back of abdomen (use back of hand), sides of abdomen <u>Hips:</u> Front, side, and back of hips <u>Lower teeth:</u> Lower teeth	<u>Pelvis, abdomen, lower teeth:</u> Place the hand over the area indicated and leave in place until release is felt. <u>Hips:</u> Place hand over the hip joint indicated and leave in place until release is felt. Alternatively, place hand on front of hip joint and move it actively in different directions until maximal softening of the indicator is felt. Hold this position until release if felt. <u>Lower back:</u> While holding your hand over the area of the abdomen indicated, bend forward, backward, and sideways, and rotate to the left and the right. Hold in the direction creating the greatest softening of the indicator until release is felt.

Condition: Hip Pain			
Description	**Common Primary Restrictions**	**Quick Tests**	**Treatment**
Hip pain may be associated with mechanical (structural) imbalance due to dysfunction in the pelvis, low back, femur (thighbone), or the hip joint itself. It may also occur due to inflammatory conditions of the pelvic organs. Hip pain that arises without any obvious strain or does not respond to self-treatment should be investigated by a health professional.	■ Pelvis ■ Low back ■ Lower abdomen ■ Hip ■ Thigh ■ Lower teeth	Pelvis: Side, front, and back of pelvis Lower back, abdomen: Front of abdomen (use palm of hand), back of abdomen (use back of hand), sides of abdomen Hips: Front, side, and back of hips Thigh: Upper, middle, and lower thigh Lower teeth: Lower teeth	Thigh: Place the hand over the area indicated and leave in place until release is felt. Also test each of the directions for mechanical treatment of long bones that creates the greatest softening of the indicator, and hold until release is felt. Pelvis, abdomen, lower teeth: Place the hand over the area indicated and leave in place until release is felt. Hips: Place hand over the hip joint indicated and leave in place until release is felt. Alternatively, place hand on front of hip joint and move it actively in different directions until maximal softening of the indicator is felt. Hold this position until release if felt. Lower back: While holding the hand over the area of the abdomen indicated, bend forward, backward, and sideways, and rotate to the left and the right. Hold in the direction creating the greatest softening of the indicator until release is felt.

Condition: Knee Pain			
Description	**Common Primary Restrictions**	**Quick Tests**	**Treatment**
Knee pain is often due to compensations for primary restrictions in the pelvis, hip, leg, or foot. It may become injured directly due to falls or severe strains. Other conditions associated with this area include leg pain and "shin splints."	■ Foot ■ Ankle ■ Knee ■ Leg ■ Thigh ■ Pelvis ■ Lower abdomen ■ Lower teeth	<u>Foot, ankle:</u> Top and bottom of foot, front, sides, and back of ankle <u>Knee:</u> Front, sides, and back of knee <u>Leg, thigh:</u> Upper, middle, and lower leg and thigh <u>Pelvis:</u> Side, front, and back of pelvis <u>Lower abdomen:</u> Front of abdomen (use palm of hand), back of abdomen (use back of hand), sides of abdomen <u>Lower teeth:</u> Lower teeth	<u>Leg, thigh:</u> Place the hand over the area indicated and leave in place until release is felt. Also test each of the directions for mechanical treatment of long bones that creates the greatest softening of the indicator and hold until release is felt. <u>Foot, ankle, knee:</u> Place the hand over the area indicated and leave in place until release is felt. Alternatively, move the joints in the direction creating the greatest softening of the indicator and hold until release is felt. <u>Pelvis, lower abdomen, lower teeth:</u> Place the hand over the area indicated and leave in place until release is felt.

Condition: Foot and Ankle Pain			
Description	**Common Primary Restrictions**	**Quick Tests**	**Treatment**
Foot and ankle pain are extremely common, often due to compensations for primary restrictions in the pelvis, hip, or leg. It may be directly due to falls or severe strains or sprains. Footwear may also affect the mechanics of the foot and corrective arch supports may be helpful. Other conditions associated with this area include plantar fasciitis, fallen arches (pronation), bunions, and Morton's neuroma.	■ Foot ■ Ankle ■ Leg ■ Pelvis ■ Lower abdomen ■ Lower teeth	Foot, ankle: Top and bottom of foot, front, sides, and back of ankle. Leg: Upper, middle, and lower leg Pelvis: Side, front, and back of pelvis Lower abdomen: Front of abdomen (use palm of hand), back of abdomen (use back of hand), sides of abdomen Lower teeth: Lower teeth	Foot, ankle: Place the hand over the area indicated and leave in place until release is felt. Alternatively, move the joints in the direction creating the greatest softening of the indicator and hold until release is felt. Leg: Place your hand over the area indicated and leave in place until release is felt. Also test each of the directions for mechanical treatment of long bones that creates the greatest softening of the indicator and hold until release is felt. Pelvis, lower abdomen, lower teeth: Place the hand over the area indicated and leave in place until release is felt.

CHAPTER 8

Keeping in Balance: The Matrix Exercise Program

The Matrix Exercise Program is designed to improve and maintain balanced muscle tone and strength, increase flexibility, and promote cardiovascular fitness. Like the Matrix Repatterning Self-Treatment Program, it works *with* the body, rather than forcing it to change. The exercise program will also support and enhance the changes you have been able to achieve in the treatment program.

It is a surprisingly simple program that utilizes nearly every muscle in the body. It is gentle, safe, and easy to do. It combines rhythmic movement, isotonic resistance, active stretching, and multiple joint mobilization components. Most of these features are combined in one basic exercise form, which can then be modified to suit a particular purpose or fitness goal.

THE PURPOSE OF EXERCISE

There are as many exercise programs as there are people with opinions about them. Most would say they feel better if they exercise in some fashion on a regular basis. Moderate cardiovascular exercise has been proven to be beneficial in reducing blood pressure, normalizing blood sugar levels and cholesterol, and reducing stress. Other forms of exercise have been advocated for general fitness, bone health, and flexibility.

Exercise has also been recommended for the management of pain or other forms of physical limitation. These are usually prescribed on the basis of some limitation in certain ranges of motion or a lack of tone or strength in one or more muscle groups. The practitioner (the physical therapist, chiropractor, doctor, or athletic trainer) typically recommends exercise to compensate for the perceived deficiency. This will usually involve specific stretches to extend the limited range of movement or to lengthen a shortened muscle or group of muscles. Other exercises are designed to strengthen areas of weakness or deficient tone. It is common knowledge that most of these efforts have only short-term benefit, and so the patient is encouraged to perform the exercises on a regular (usually daily) basis. The patient may experience some benefit if the exercises are performed regularly but usually experiences a return of symptoms if the program is interrupted.

One of the goals of Matrix Repatterning is to restore optimal function to the entire structure of the body. Therefore, the need for exercise to correct imbalances in the joints or muscles becomes unnecessary. The purpose of the Matrix Exercise Program is to enhance strength, tone, and overall flexibility in the structure of the body and to promote increased cardiovascular efficiency. It is not designed nor intended to compensate for imbalances in function, as this can be gently and effectively accomplished through Matrix Repatterning treatments. Once relative balance is achieved, muscles and joints will function more efficiently and with less tendency to become strained. Therefore, efforts to increase strength and tone in muscle can be accomplished more easily. Flexibility appears to be dependent on intracellular and extracellular alignment of the molecules that make up the matrix and connect one cell to another. The Total Body Stretch addresses the need for optimal flexibility through a gentle, coordinated approach.

THE EXERCISE PROGRAM

There are three components to the program: the Circular Push, the Circular Pull, and the Total Body Stretch.

The Circular Push

The circular push and the next exercise (circular pull) consist of a standing posture with the hands held in front of the body. A similar approach may also be accomplished in a seated position. Stand with the feet positioned at shoulder width. The hands are placed palm to palm near the center of the chest. Turn slowly at the hips, allowing the foot on the opposite side from the direction you are turning to pivot on the ball of the foot. At the same time push your hands gently together. Feel the rotation through the abdomen and hips and gently hold the abdominal muscles in, providing slight resistance against the turning movement. Be aware of the increase in tension in the thigh and hip muscles, and accentuate these slightly in order to push into the turn. In the upper body, create a slight resistance through the hands and arms against the turning motion. Repeat this action in the opposite direction and continue the rotations from side to side until you have completed your desired number of repetitions.

The overall effect is like one half of your body is pushing into the turn, while the other half is trying to resist the movement. Let the side of the body that is pushing win, but give it a good workout in the process. This isotonic (equal force) resistance provides the toning component of the exercise. As the resistance and speed of the turns are increased, an effective cardiovascular effect is also achieved.

Three sets of pushes may be performed with the arms in a mid-body position, a lower body position (in front of the pelvis) and in an upper body position (in front of the head). Each position exercises different muscle groups and joints.

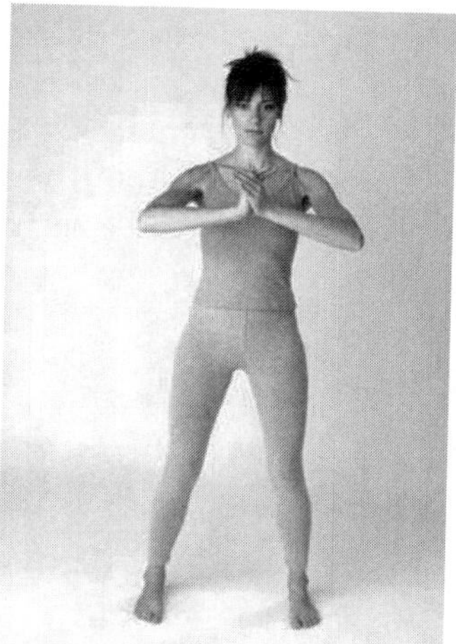
Figure 8-1: Circular push mid-body starting position

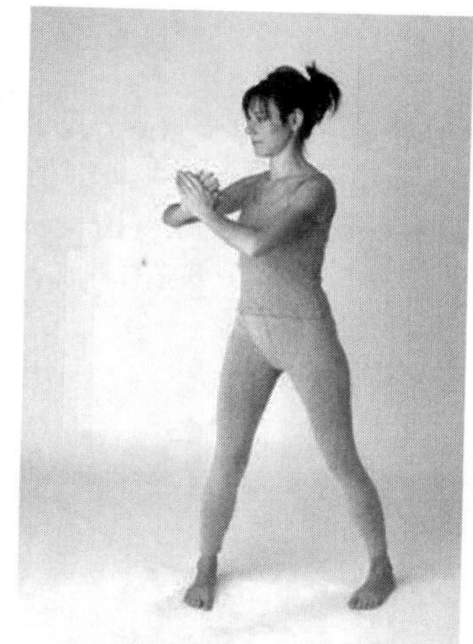
Figure 8-2: Circular push right

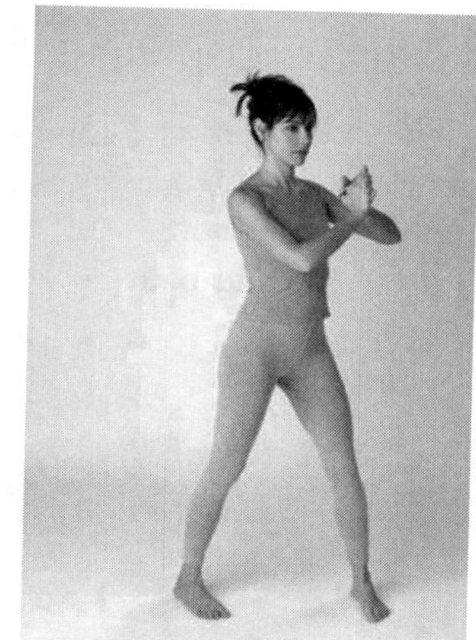
Figure 8-3: Circular push left

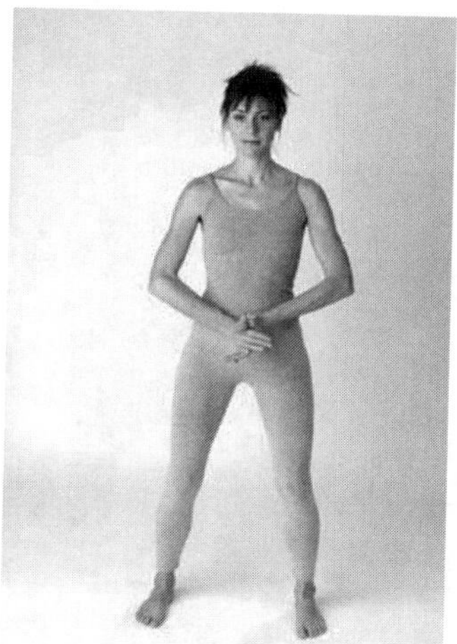
Figure 8-4: Circular push lower body starting position

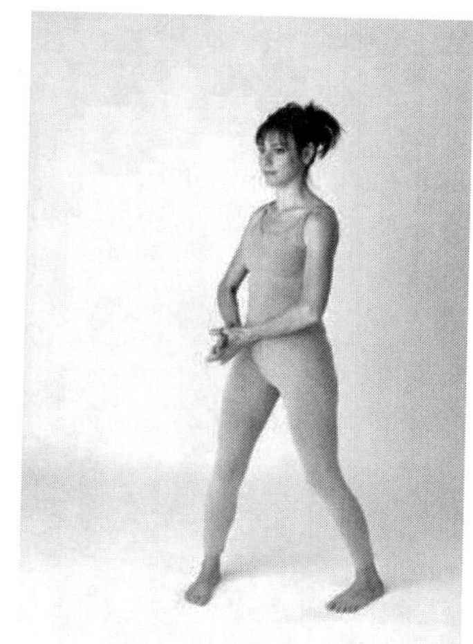
Figure 8-5: Circular push right

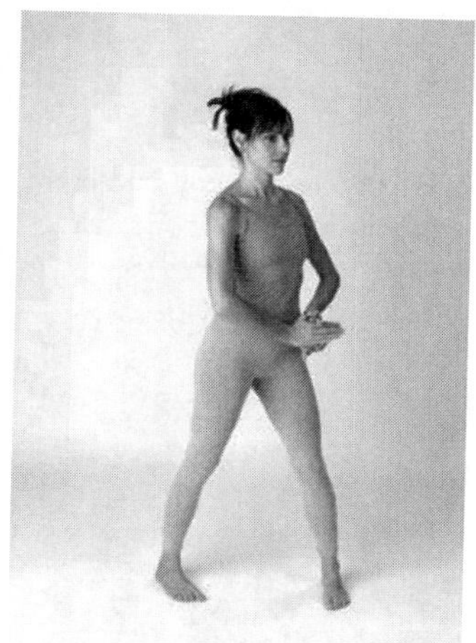
Figure 8-6: Circular push left

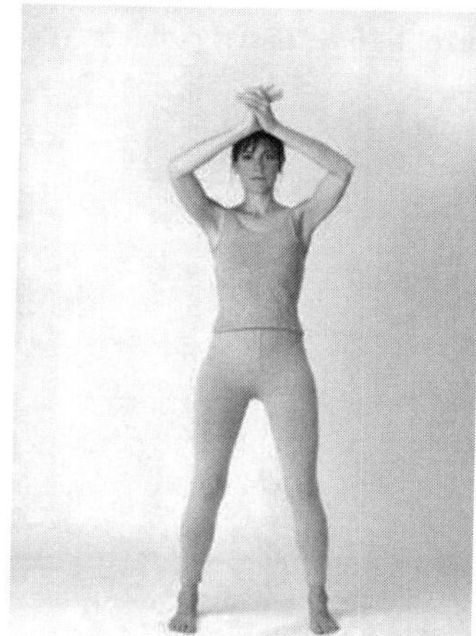
Figure 8-7: Circular push upper body starting position

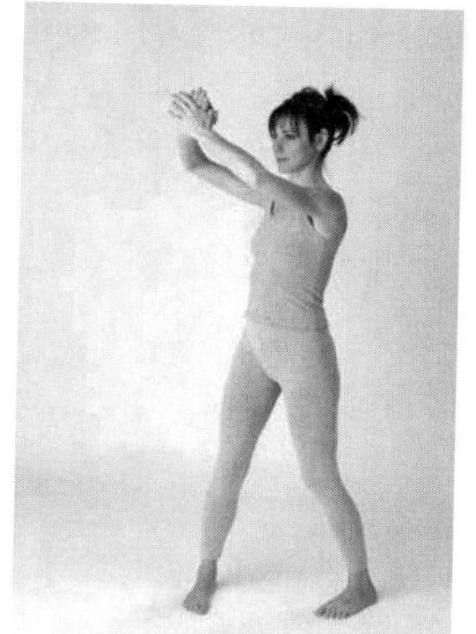
Figure 8-8: Circular push right

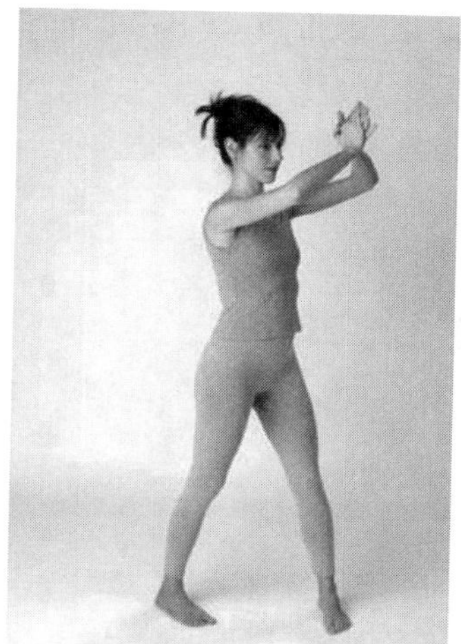
Figure 8-9: Circular push left

The Circular Pull

The stance for the circular pull is the same as for the circular push. In this exercise, however, the resistance to turning is done by pulling the hands apart, with the side of the body away from the turn attempting—but failing—to prevent the turning motion. This series is also composed of three sets with the arms in the mid-body, lower body, and upper body positions.

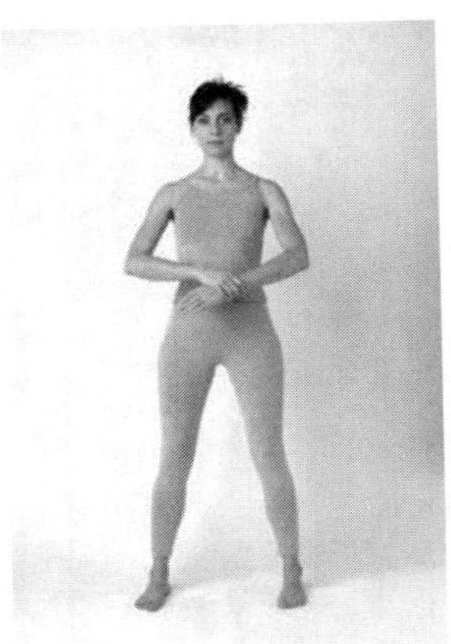

Figure 8-10: Circular pull mid-body starting position

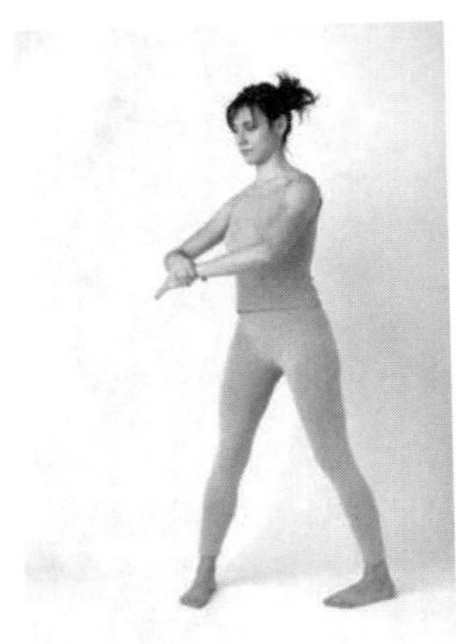

Figure 8-11: Circular pull right

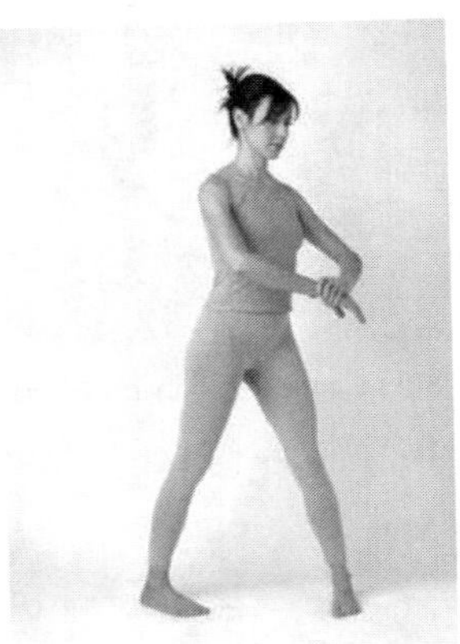

Figure 8-12: Circular pull left

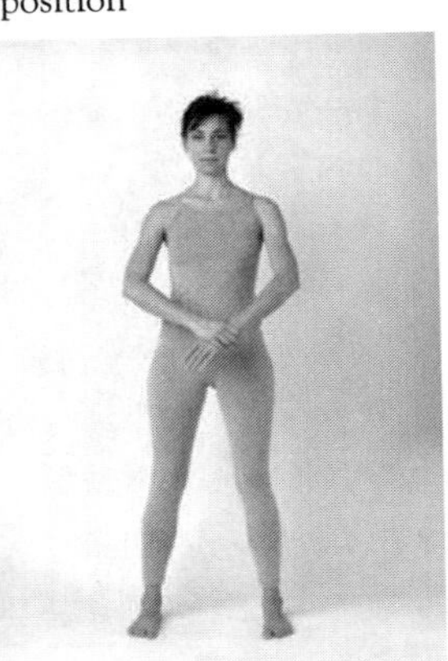

Figure 8-13: Circular pull lower body starting position

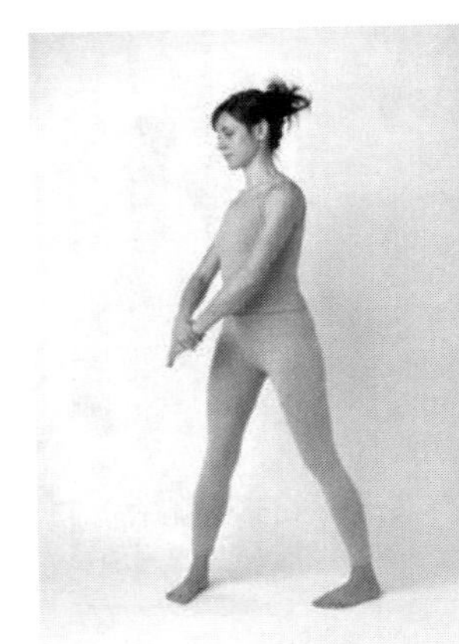

Figure 8-14: Circular pull right

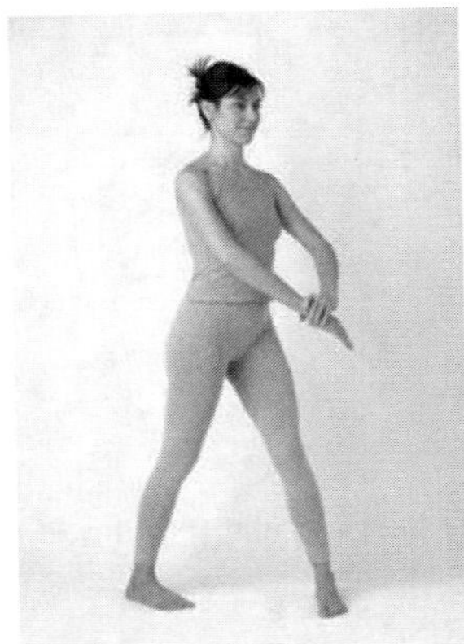

Figure 8-15: Circular pull left

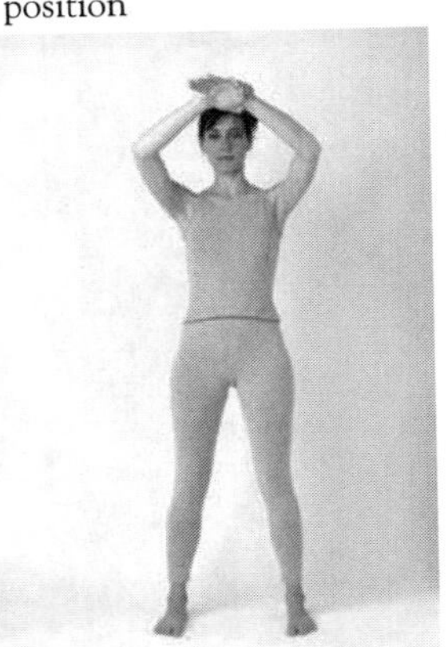

Figure 8-16: Circular pull upper body starting position

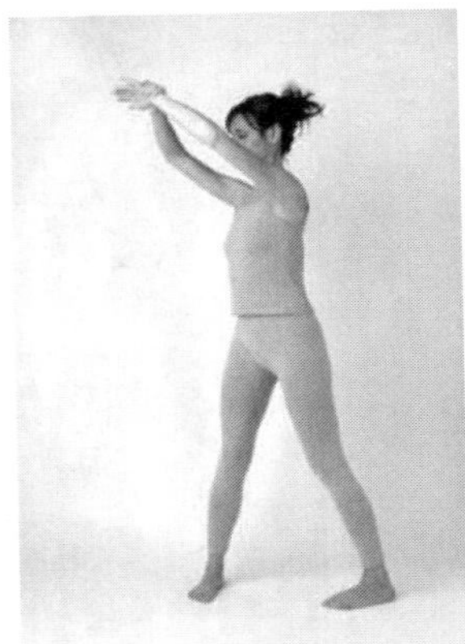

Figure 8-17: Circular pull right

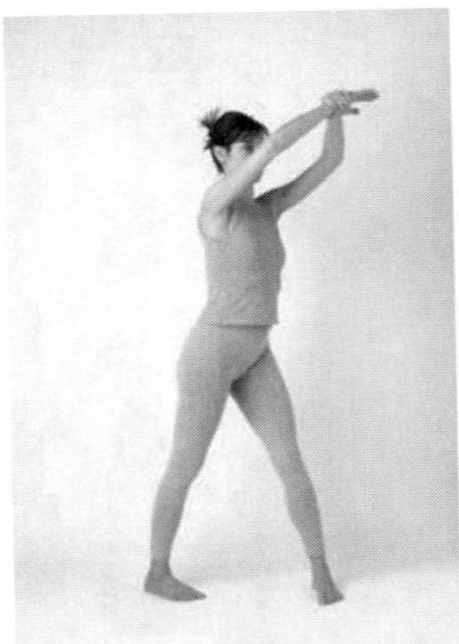

Figure 8-18: Circular pull left

The Total Body Stretch

Stretching as a form of therapy has often been used to compensate for tension patterns created by primary restrictions. The problem is that when stretching is used to release areas of tension, it is usually the tissues around the primary restrictions, which are more flexible, that will tend to give more. Therefore, it may appear that the tense area is being lengthened, when in reality it is only that the surrounding tissues are being overstretched. In fact, due to the characteristics of the matrix, the more forcefully you stretch, the less likely it is that you will actually release the restricted area. This is due to the electrical properties of the matrix, which resist forceful deformation.

Once an area has been in a restricted state for a long period of time, the water molecules become displaced and the result may be a shortened condition of the tissues (Pollack 2001). The purpose of stretching, ideally, is to open the molecular framework in order to allow water molecules to be drawn into the area and re-establish their position around the protein elements of the matrix. This process restores the ideal volume and flexibility to the area.

In its ideal healthy state, the tensegrity matrix requires very little to maintain its perfectly balanced functional characteristics. It has been the experience of many, including world-class athletes, that rigorous stretching becomes much less of a requirement for optimal performance once they are structurally balanced through the Matrix Repatterning Program.

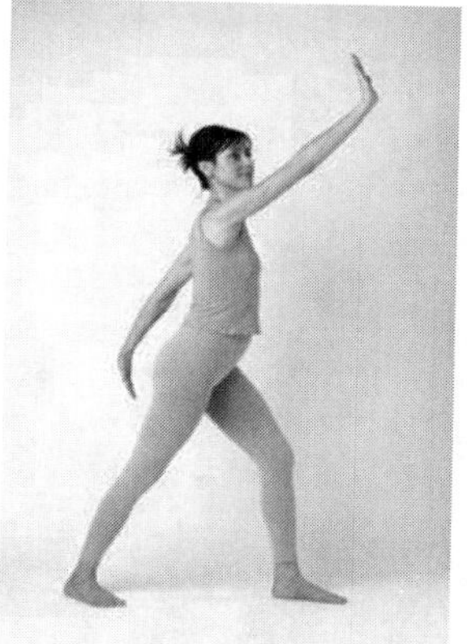

Figure 8-19: Cross stretch right

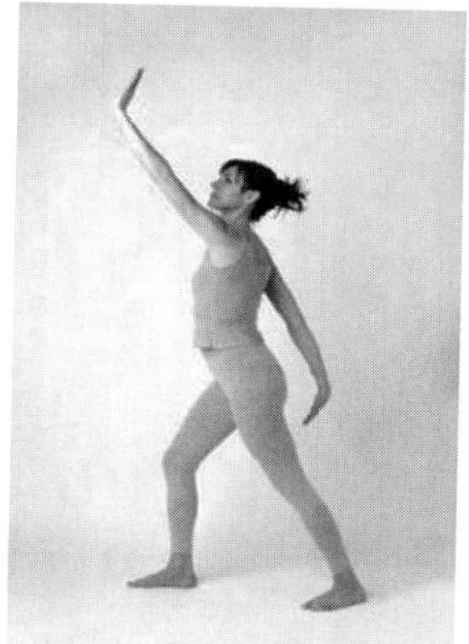

Figure 8-20: Cross stretch left

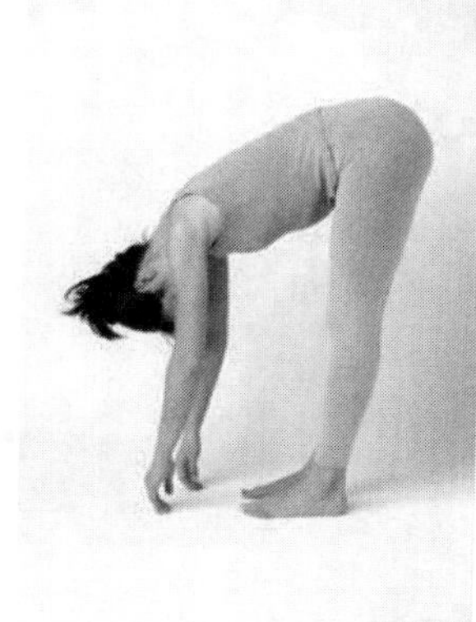

Figure 8-21: Forward stretch

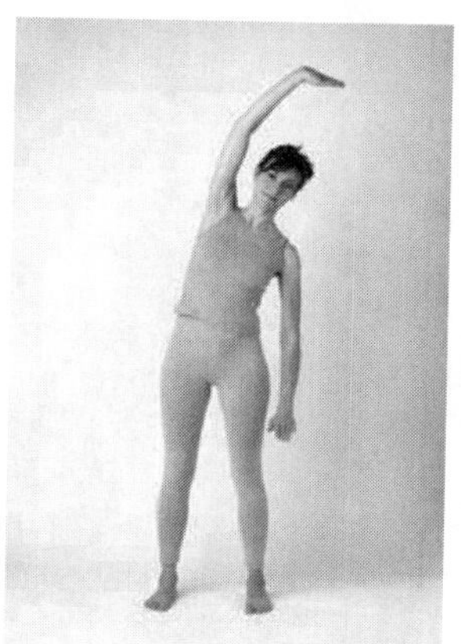

Figure 8-22: Side stretch right

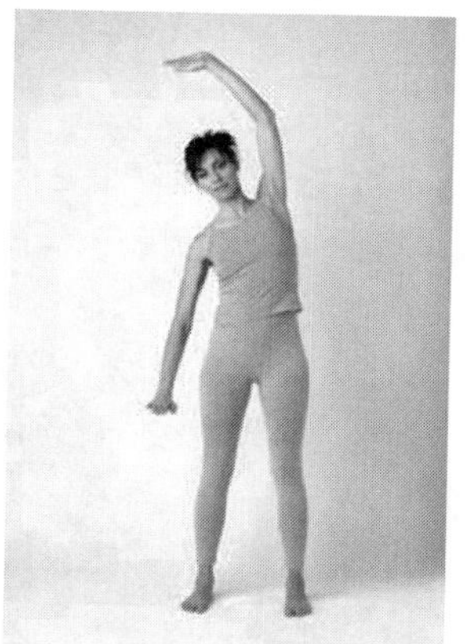

Figure 8-23: Side stretch left

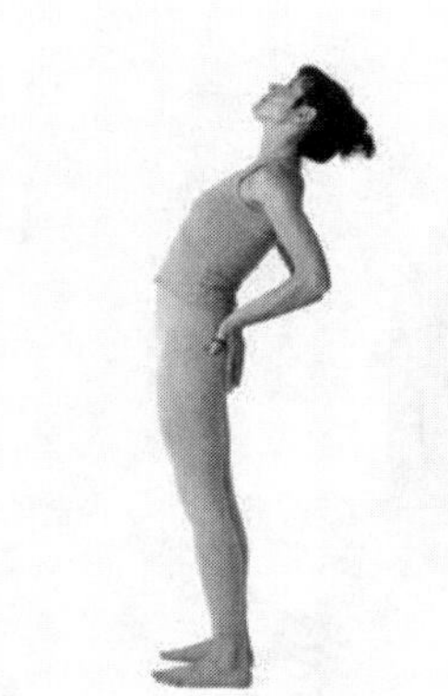

Figure 8-24: Backward stretch

The Matrix Exercise Program should be an enjoyable experience. Use it as an opportunity to appreciate your body, feeling its strength, resilience, and vitality. As you perform the exercises, be aware of your breathing and the flow of energy in different areas as you release tension gently and comfortably.

As you progress in your quest to achieve optimal health and freedom from pain through the Matrix Repatterning Program, you will find that the exercises will become more and more invigorating and energizing. You may find that you look forward to using your body in other enjoyable ways, perhaps through sports activities and with various recreational and fun outdoor activities.

It is my belief that you will achieve your goal of becoming pain free through the methods described in this book. It is also my hope that you can enjoy a higher level of well-being and optimal health by restoring balance to the structure of your body through Matrix Repatterning.

APPENDIX I

The Matrix Repatterning Experience

As mentioned throughout the book, you may run into problems that the self-treatment techniques don't quite resolve. In these cases, you should seek out a Matrix Repatterning practitioner (see appendix 3). This section presents an overview of a Matrix Repatterning session as performed by a professional practitioner. Individual practitioners may vary certain aspects of this procedure.

HEALTH HISTORY

The Matrix Repatterning practitioner first takes a careful health history to determine the nature of your symptoms or other limitations, including any injuries and surgeries. This will guide the practitioner in determining what tests may need to be performed in order to rule out other potentially serious illnesses that may be contributing to your situation.

STRUCTURAL ASSESSMENT

This assessment may include an examination of your posture, ranges of motion, muscle tone, nervous system responses, and other tests to determine any abnormalities or differences from one side of the body to the other. These tests are important since they can provide an objective basis for determining the effectiveness of treatment. Changes in your symptoms, although they may improve noticeably, may take some time to resolve. It is important for the practitioner—and for you—to have objectively measurable indicators of change in order to determine how your body is responding to treatment.

LOCATING THE SOURCE

The Matrix Repatterning practitioner will test the flexibility of the rib cage, the shoulder, a muscle, or another part of the body while contacting a series of locations throughout the body. These areas used to test other areas of the body are referred to as *indicators*. This is because they are used to indicate a source of tension somewhere else in the body. The molecular restriction is in fact an electrical disturbance in which the force of an injury has altered the molecular state. A normal electrical field placed near the disturbed field will tend to shift it toward normal. This property of electromagnetic fields is referred to as *entrainment*. Therefore, when the practitioner places his or her hand over an area of primary restriction, it will temporarily be reduced. Because the tensegrity matrix is interconnected throughout the body, the entire body will relax slightly. This is a response the practitioner can readily detect and it can usually be felt by the patient.

The purpose of the assessment is to locate the sources of molecular tension (referred to as *primary restrictions*) in the body. This process is continued until all of the restrictions are detected and noted. The practitioner will then determine the priority in which these areas are to be treated.

TREATMENT: MINIMAL FORCE AT THE SOURCE

A primary restriction is created by energy or force being trapped inside the molecules, causing the area to become rigid and restricted—hence the term "restriction." This causes an increase in the local electrical charge within the tissues of the body that have been injured. Treatment is intended to release this excess charge in order to encourage the matrix to return to its natural relaxed and flexible state. Matrix Repatterning treatment usually consists of placing a hand over the area of restriction. The hands produce a normal electrical field that can influence the injured area to return to normal. This property of electrical fields, as mentioned earlier, is called entrainment and helps to release the trapped electrical energy in the area. This may be why we instinctively place our own hands over an area right after an injury.

The Matrix Repatterning practitioner will also usually add some pressure into the part being treated. This has the effect of increasing the movement of the electrical charge. The pressure is applied very precisely and gently to coax or encourage these areas to discharge the built-up electrical charge maintaining the restriction. The patient often feels a release of tension in the area as this static charge is converted to moving electrons, which is actually a form of electrical current.

Treatments are very gentle. The reason they can be performed with minimal force is that the instrument doing the work, the practitioner's hand, provides a normalizing influence in harmony with the tissues being treated. On occasion, an electronic device may be used. These devices produce an electrical signal with similar properties to the current produced by the body. This is helpful in areas that are inflamed or affected by scar tissue, where the normal electrical field has been seriously compromised (Biedebach 1989).

The changes created by treatment tend to be long-lasting, since the molecules have been returned to a more stable configuration. Unless another significant injury or energy input is sustained, the pattern of tension will not return. Each area may need to be treated in several slightly different directions in order to release the entire pattern. Several primary areas may be treated in any one session.

RESTORING THE PATTERN

The actual release may be accomplished by gentle pressure against the resistance of the restriction patterns. This process may take several minutes and is referred to as *induction*. During this time the patient may experience a building of pressure in the area being treated. Although Matrix Repatterning is generally relaxing and painless, occasionally symptoms such as pain, a sensation of heat or burning, and vibration may occur. Another method of treatment involves *directional recoil*. This involves placing pressure over the primary restriction, but instead of holding the area, the practitioner will suddenly release the pressure. It is believed that this sudden, gentle springing motion creates an oscillation within the tissues. This could be compared to a medical device called a *defibrillator*, which is used in conventional medicine to restore the normal electrical pattern to an irregularly beating heart. The defibrillator generates an electrical charge similar in pattern to that created by the heart but much larger in magnitude. Directional recoil and induction may cause the excess electrical charge stored within the restricted area of the tensegrity matrix to dissipate. The result of this process is that the treated tissues relax and normal tone is re-established.

ADAPTING TO CHANGE

Since practitioners are often addressing long-term imbalances, the body may react for a period of several days after treatments. This is especially true after the first few sessions, since larger, more significant restrictions are usually being addressed. As these larger patterns, which may have been in place for many months or years, are released, the change in the overall state of tension is greater, and therefore the body experiences a more significant relative difference from the previous state. Some discomfort may occur and old symptoms may resurface as the body reorganizes itself toward a new state of balance.

LAYERING: THE ARCHEOLOGY OF RELEASING TRAUMA

The tensegrity matrix can dissipate most day-to-day bumps and strains, which will therefore have no lasting effect. The higher the energy imparted to the tissues, the greater the number of molecules and cells that will be shifted toward the high-energy, restricted state. Thus, a significant incident will affect a larger area and cause more energy to be absorbed by the body than a less significant event.

Each tension pattern is thus associated with a sort of energetic signature directly proportional to the magnitude of the injury or other source of energy input. A primary restriction with a large energy signature will tend to overshadow other patterns with smaller energy signatures and will therefore be more obvious, from a diagnostic perspective, compared to less significant patterns. In this way, tension or strain patterns will be revealed in an order of priority directly related to the amount of energy trapped within the tissues. Many less significant patterns will actually be diagnostically invisible until restrictions of a higher order are released. As the more significant primary restrictions are released, the patterns with smaller energy signatures will become evident. This could be compared to an archeological expedition, as layer after layer of injury patterns are revealed. In this way, all of the structural imbalances developed over a lifetime can be revealed and released through a series of treatments.

APPENDIX 2

Home Care Measures

The recommendations in this section are to provide you with simple measures to facilitate the restoration of structural balance, to reduce inflammation and pain, and to optimize the benefits you achieve from the Matrix Repatterning Program.

CASTOR OIL COMPRESS: SELF-TREATMENT FOR SCAR TISSUE

Castor oil has been shown to increase circulation and promote elimination in the organs and tissues. It stimulates lymph circulation and increases the levels of certain white blood cells that are involved in the removal of toxins and inflammatory debris (McGarey 1999). This can aid in the reduction of pain and swelling and help improve flexibility by reducing adhesions and scar tissue.

The compress may be placed over an inflamed area that is not an open wound. This may be an old surgical site or a chronically inflamed or arthritic joint.

Materials

- Castor oil (cold-pressed)
- Small glass pan
- White flannel cloth (folded to achieve 2 to 3 thicknesses), enough to cover the affected area

- Hot water bottle
- Plastic wrap or small plastic bag

Method

1. Pour a small quantity of castor oil in the pan.
2. Soak the flannel in the castor oil.
3. Heat the soaked flannel in the glass pan gently on a stove until warm, or warm in a microwave oven.
4. Place the flannel on the affected area.
5. Cover with a plastic sheet.
6. Place a hot water bottle or heated towel over the plastic sheet and leave in place for 60 minutes.
7. The compress may be left in place for another 1 to 2 hours, or overnight.
8. Rest while the compress is in place.
9. After removal of the compress, cleanse the area with water or with a thin paste made of water and baking soda combined in a mixture.
10. The compress should be stored in a covered container in the refrigerator and may be reused several times. It should be discarded if it begins to show signs of rancidity.
11. Apply the compress no more than 5 times per week for 1 to 3 weeks.

COLD THERAPY

Using ice to treat injuries is one of the oldest methods of pain control. Proven to be safe and effective at reducing swelling, relieving pain, and decreasing muscle spasms, ice therapy is an easy self-care technique that anyone can administer. Cold therapy, also known as *cryotherapy*, works on the principle of heat exchange. This occurs when you place a cooler object in direct contact with an object of warmer temperature, such as ice against skin. The cooler object will absorb the heat of the warmer object. Why is this important when it comes to cold therapy?

After an injury, blood vessels that deliver oxygen and nutrients to cells are damaged. The cells around the injury then increase their metabolism, thus consuming more oxygen. When all of the oxygen is used up, the cells die. Also, the damaged blood vessels cannot remove waste. Blood cells and fluid seep into spaces around the muscle, resulting in swelling and bruising. When ice is applied, it lowers the temperature of the damaged tissue through heat exchange and constricts local blood vessels. This slows the cells' metabolism and the consumption of oxygen, therefore reducing the rate of cell damage and decreasing fluid build-up. Ice can also numb nerve endings. This stops the transfer of impulses to the brain that register as pain.

Most therapists and doctors advise not to use heat right after an injury, as this will have the opposite effect of ice. Heat increases blood flow and relaxes muscles. It's good for easing tight muscles but will only increase the pain and swelling of an injury by accelerating metabolism.

Different cooling methods will produce different effects due to the device's ability to exchange heat. Crushed ice packs do a better job at cooling the body than chemical or gel packs because they last longer and are able to draw four times the amount of heat out of tissue. The important difference is that ice packs undergo phase change from ice to water, allowing them to maintain an even temperature for a longer period, creating a more effective treatment. Most chemical or one-time-use packs and gel packs do not undergo this type of phase change. They quickly lose their ability to transfer heat, limiting their effectiveness in reducing swelling. Their short duration of cold is not long enough to produce numbness, also reducing their ability to relieve pain.

Cold therapy should always be used as soon as possible after an injury occurs and continued for the following forty-eight hours. It should be applied for no longer than ten minutes at a time, using shorter intervals for smaller parts of the body. For example, your finger will lose heat more quickly than your thigh. Each cooling interval should be followed by an equal interval without cold to allow the circulation to nourish the area and remove wastes. The cooling and noncooling intervals should be repeated approximately three to four times every one to two hours.

EPSOM SALTS BATHS

Epsom salts are composed of magnesium sulfate. Magnesium is an important factor in muscle contractility. The benefits of immersing the body in a bath containing Epsom salts may be due to the magnesium content and its muscle-relaxing effects. The effect of heat may also enhance the effects of the bath, which can increase vasodilatation, local circulation, metabolism, and overall relaxation. An Epsom salt bath may also help to reduce pain and muscle spasm.

The temperature of the bath should be no higher than 100 degrees Fahrenheit (38° C), and duration may be up to fifteen minutes.

Method

1. Add 1 to 2 cups (250 to 500 cc) of Epsom salts to the bathwater.
2. Stay in the bath for a minimum of 5 minutes and a maximum of 15 minutes.
3. Take a cool shower to rinse off the Epsom salts.

AVOIDING ELECTRICAL IMBALANCE

Several scientific studies have pointed to a correlation between exposure to certain types of electromagnetic fields and the development of certain diseases, including cancer (Liburdy et al. 1993; Burr 1972).

The tensegrity matrix has very specific electromagnetic properties, and so it makes sense that it might become influenced by external fields, especially if it is compromised structurally.

The increase in the development of electronic devices in this technological age has been a boon to the economy and a potential minefield to the health of the individual. These devices include cell phones, pagers, computer monitors, and various electrical appliances. We have been exposed to increasing levels of various forms of artificially produced electromagnetic fields with very little understanding of their short- or long-term health effects.

Based on the Matrix Repatterning assessment, it is evident that certain types of devices produce fields that tend to negatively influence the molecular structure of the body. Using the indicator (as described in chapter 4) can easily test this. Simply place yourself in proximity to the electrical device, such as a cell phone or computer and test the indicator. Turn off the device or remove yourself at least four feet from the device and retest. If the field is affecting you in a negative way, the indicator will become firm or more resistant when you're near the device.

Manufacturers of electronic devices are becoming more aware of the potential health hazards associated with these devices and have taken steps to reduce or alter the fields to render them less damaging. Therefore, newer devices may be more easily tolerated by the body than older ones. For example, computer screens have been altered in recent years to reduce their electromagnetic emissions. Interestingly, this field has been reduced only at the front of the screen. The sides, top, and back of the standard cathode-ray screens still produce strong electromagnetic fields.

The issue of metal in close contact with the body has also become a concern. In a sense, it may be compared to placing a piece of metal in a circuit board. Therefore, it may be a problem for some people if they wear items that include metal, such as brassieres with metal underwires or watches with metal watchbands. Smaller items such as rings and earrings tend to be less problematic.

The earth naturally produces a strong magnetic field associated with the magnetic polarity of the planet. Since our body also has a directional magnetic field (Oschman 2000), it has been found that some individuals are sensitive to the direction in which they spend a large portion of time in relation to the earth's magnetic field. You may find, for example, that if you have difficulty falling asleep or difficulty achieving deeper levels of sleep or if you awaken feeling unrested or in pain, that you are sensitive to these directional factors. In general, the human body seems to function better when the sleeping position is such that the head points toward the north or the east. If in doubt, use an indicator to determine the best direction for yourself.

APPENDIX 3

Finding a Matrix Repatterning Practitioner

SELF-TREATMENT WORKSHOPS

Self-Treatment Workshops are being planned for different regions throughout the world. These are presented by certified Matrix Repatterning Self-Treatment facilitators and are designed to provide you with assistance in developing the skills you need to become proficient in the application of the principles presented in this book. For information on locations, dates, and costs, please contact us at the address below.

HOW TO FIND A MATRIX REPATTERNING PRACTITIONER

Matrix Repatterning practitioners include professionals such as physical therapists, sports-medicine specialists, chiropractors, osteopaths, physiatrists, massage therapists, athletic trainers, and others. Training in Matrix Repatterning is available to students and graduates of these programs throughout North America, in Europe, and in Central America.

The training program involves extensive theoretic and practical seminars, as well as evaluation and certification of clinical proficiency. Once completed, the practitioner is conferred with a certificate in Matrix Repatterning. Before certification, the practitioner may elect to incorporate some aspects of the technique into their practice. Since there are no contraindications to its use, meaning there are no risks to the patient, this is a valid approach and is one that allows the practitioner to gradually increase their skills while providing a very real benefit to the patient.

Certification involves a more detailed and extensive training program, as well as the successful completion of a proficiency examination by a M.R. instructor. This certification essentially provides the public with a guideline to choosing a practitioner with an assured level of skill and training in this technique.

The names of certified practitioners and others who have completed advanced training (pre-certification) are available by contacting us at the address listed below.

Contact Information:

The Roth Institute (a division of Wellness Systems Inc.)
P.O. Box 1
Newmarket, Ontario Canada L3Y 4W3
Web site: www.rothinstitute.com
E-mail: info@rothinstitute.com

References

Biedebach, M. 1989. Accelerated healing of skin ulcers by electrical stimulation and the intracellular physiological mechanisms involved. *Acupuncture and Electro-Therapeutics Research, International Journal* 19:43-60.

Burr, H. S. 1972. *Blueprint for Immortality: The Electrical Patterns of Life.* London: Neville Spearman.

D'Ambrogio, K., and G. Roth. 1997. *Positional Release Therapy: Assessment & Treatment of Musculoskeletal Dysfunction.* St. Louis: Elsevier (Harcourt-Mosby).

Denslow, J. S., I. M. Korr, and A. B. Krems. 1947. Quantitative studies of chronic facilitation in human motoneuron pools. *American Journal of Physiology* 150:229.

Dienstfrey, H. 1991. *Where the Mind Meet the Body: Type A, the Relaxation Response, Psychoneuroimmunology, Biofeedback, Neuropeptides, Hypnosis, Imagery and the Search for the Mind's Effects on Physical Health.* New York: HarperCollins.

Duncan, R. L. 1995. Transduction of mechanical strain in bone. *Gravitational and Space Biology Bulletin* 8:49-62.

Feynman, R. 1974. *Surely You're Joking, Mr. Feynman!* Edited by Edward Hutchings. New York: W. W. Norton.

Fingerhut, L. A., and M. Warner. 1997. *Injury Chartbook: Healthy United States, 1996-97.* Hyattsville, MD: National Center for Health Statistics.

Gould, L. 1984. Magnetic field sensitivity in animals. *Annual Review of Physiology* 46:585-598.

Hatfaludy, S., J. Hannsky, and H. H. Vandenburgh. 1989. Metabolic alterations induced in cultured skeletal muscle by stretch-relaxation activity. *American Journal of Physiology* 256:C175-181.

Hawley, C. A. 2004. Outcomes following childhood head injury: A popular study. *Journal of Neurology, Neurosurgery, and Psychiatry.*

H'Doubler, F. 1994. Treatment of post-polio syndrome with electro-stimulation of auricular acupuncture points: An evaluation of twelve patients. *American Journal of Acupuncture* 22(1):15-21.

Heidemann, S. R. 1993. A new twist on integrins and the cytoskeleton. *Science* 260:1080-1081.

Ingber, D. E. 1998. The architecture of life. *Scientific American* 278:48-57.

———. 2002. Mechanical signaling and the cellular response to extracellular matrix in angiogenesis and cardiovascular physiology. *Circulatory Research* 91:877-887.

———. 2003. Mechanobiology and diseases of mechanotransduction. *Annals of Medicine* 35:1-14.

Ko, K. S., P. D. Arora, and C. A. McCulloch. 2001. Cadherins mediate intercellular mechanicl signaling in fibroblasts by activation of stretch-sensitive-calcium-permeable channels. *Journal of Biological Chemistry* 276:35967-35977.

Levin, S. M. 2002. The tensegrity-truss as a model for spine mechanics. *Journal of Mechanics in Medicine Biology* 2:375-388.

Lewitt, K. 1985. The muscular and articular factor in movement restriction. *Manual Medicine* 1:83-85.

Liburdy, R. P., T. R. Sloan, R. Sokolic, and P. Yaswen. 1993. ELF magnetic fields, breast cancer, and melatonin: 60HZ fields block melatonin's oncostatic action on ER+ breast cancer cell proliferation. *Journal of Pineal Research* 14(2):89-97.

Marsland, D. A., and D. E. S. Brown. 1942. The effects of pressure on sol-gel equilibria, with special reference to myosin and other protoplasmic gels. *Journal of Cellular and Comparative Physiology* 20:295-305.

Masi, A. T., and E. G. Walsh. 2003. Ankylosing spondylitis: Integrated clinical and physiological perspectives. *Clinical Experimental Rheumatology* 21:1-8.

McGarey, W. A. 1999. *The Oil That Heals: A Physician's Successes with Castor Oil Treatments.* Viginia Beach: A.R.E. Press.

Moseley, J. B., K. O'Malley, N. J. Petersen, T. J. Menke, B. A. Brody, D. H. Kuykendall, J. C. Hollingsworth, C. M. Ashton, and N. P. Wray. 2002. A controlled trial of arthroscopic surgery for osteoarthritis of the knee. *New England Journal of Medicine* 347(2):81-88

National Institutes of Heath. 1985. *Injury in America: A Continuing Public Health Problem.* Washington D.C.: National Academy Press.

Oschman, J. L. 2000. *Energy Medicine: The Scientific Basis.* London: Churchill Livingstone.

Oschman, J. L., and N. H. Oschman. 1994. Physiological and emotional effects of acupuncture needle insertion. Paper presented at the second symposioum of the Society for Acupuncture Research, Washington, D.C.

Pert, C. B. 1997. *Molecules of Emotion.* New York: Touchstone.

Pollack, G. H. 2001. *Cells, Gels and the Engines of Life: A New Unifying Approach to Cell Function.* Seattle: Ebner & Sons.

Rachlin, E. 1994. *Myofascial Pain and Fibromyalgia.* St. Louis: Mosby.

Roth, G. B. 2000. A new approach to frozen shoulder: A pilot study using Matrix Repatterning. Second Annual Conference of Canadian Chiropractic Research Centers. Toronto.

Sarno, J. E. 1982. *Mind Over Back Pain.* New York: Berkley.

———. 1991. *Healing Back Pain: The Mind-Body Connection.* New York: Warner Books.

Seto, A., C. Kusaka, S. Nakazato, W. R. Hwang, T. Sato, T. Hisamitsu, and C. Takeshige. 1992. Detection of extraordinary large bio-magnetic field strength from human hand during external Qi emission. *Acupuncture and Electro-Therapeutics Research* 17:75-94.

Szent-Gyorgyi, Albert. 1977. "Drive in Living Matter to Perfect Itself," *Synthesis 1,* Vol. 1, No. 1, pp. 14-26.

Tanaka, T. 1981. Gels. *Scientific American* 244:124-138.

Wall, P. 2000. *The Science of Pain and Suffering.* London: Weidenfeld and Nicholson.

Wang, N., J. P. Butler, and D. E. Ingber. 1993. Mechanotransduction across the cell surface and through the cytoskeleton. *Science* 260:1124-1127.

Waylonis, G. W., and R. H. Perkins. 1994. Post-traumatic fibromyalgia. A long-term follow-up. *American Journal of Physical Medicine and Rehabilitation* 73(6):403-412.

Zimmerman, J. 1990. Laying-on-of-hands healing and therapeutic touch: A testable theory. *BEMI Currents, Journal of the Bio-Electro-Magnetics Institute* 2:8-17.

George Roth, DC, ND, is a chiropractor and naturopathic physician. He teaches seminars to health professionals and the public on general health and disease prevention. He specializes in the rehabilitation of musculoskeletal conditions and has acted as a consultant to sports injury clinics and professional athletes. He has published articles in several professional journals and has presented his research to medical audiences throughout North America. He is the coauthor of *Positional Release Therapy*.

Roth is in private practice in the Toronto area. He has two sons and is a sailing and scuba diving enthusiast. Visit Dr. Roth online at **www.matrixrepatterning.com.**

Foreword writer **James L. Oschman, Ph.D.,** is president of Nature's Own Research Association. He has degrees in biophysics and biology from the University of Pittsburgh and has worked in major research labs at Cambridge University, Case-Western Reserve University, the University of Copenhagen, Northwestern University, and the Marine Biological Laboratory in Woods Hole, MA. He is past president of the New England School of Acupuncture and holds a Distinguished Service Award from the Rolf Institute. He continues his research and writing in Dover, NH.

Some Other New Harbinger Titles

Eating Mindfully, Item 3503, $13.95
Living with RSDS, Item 3554 $16.95
The Ten Hidden Barriers to Weight Loss, Item 3244 $11.95
The Sjogren's Syndrome Survival Guide, Item 3562 $15.95
Stop Feeling Tired, Item 3139 $14.95
Responsible Drinking, Item 2949 $18.95
The Mitral Valve Prolapse/Dysautonomia Survival Guide, Item 3031 $14.95
Stop Worrying Abour Your Health, Item 285X $14.95
The Vulvodynia Survival Guide, Item 2914 $15.95
The Multifidus Back Pain Solution, Item 2787 $12.95
Move Your Body, Tone Your Mood, Item 2752 $17.95
The Chronic Illness Workbook, Item 2647 $16.95
Coping with Crohn's Disease, Item 2655 $15.95
The Woman's Book of Sleep, Item 2493 $14.95
The Trigger Point Therapy Workbook, Item 2507 $19.95
Fibromyalgia and Chronic Myofascial Pain Syndrome, second edition, Item 2388 $19.95
Kill the Craving, Item 237X $18.95
Rosacea, Item 2248 $13.95
Thinking Pregnant, Item 2302 $13.95
Shy Bladder Syndrome, Item 2272 $13.95
Help for Hairpullers, Item 2329 $13.95
Coping with Chronic Fatigue Syndrome, Item 0199 $13.95
The Stop Smoking Workbook, Item 0377 $17.95
Multiple Chemical Sensitivity, Item 173X $16.95
Breaking the Bonds of Irritable Bowel Syndrome, Item 1888 $14.95
Parkinson's Disease and the Art of Moving, Item 1837 $16.95
The Addiction Workbook, Item 0431 $18.95
The Interstitial Cystitis Survival Guide, Item 2108 $15.95

Call **toll free, 1-800-748-6273,** or log on to our online bookstore at **www.newharbinger.com** to order. Have your Visa or Mastercard number ready. Or send a check for the titles you want to New Harbinger Publications, Inc., 5674 Shattuck Ave., Oakland, CA 94609. Include $4.50 for the first book and 75¢ for each additional book, to cover shipping and handling. (California residents please include appropriate sales tax.) Allow two to five weeks for delivery.

Prices subject to change without notice.